For Scott
for always, always believing in me

and

For Betty

Table of Contents

Prologue
The Red Shoe Box

I picked up a red shoe box at the bottom of an old suitcase. My nose wrinkled as I blew the thin layer of dust off the lid, the dust motes dancing in the afternoon light streaming through my bedroom window. I lifted the lid enjoying the anticipation of discovery. I was nine again, searching for buried treasure.

Scott and I were moving. I was going through boxes of my things, sifting through memories, deeming what was to be in the keep or throw-away pile. I had no trouble throwing things out, not being one for clutter. This time was different. I don't know if it was that I was thirty-four and feeling considerably more grown up, or that I had just not looked through these boxes in years and needed to remember. But I found myself placing my hands on the past, wrapping myself around a long time ago.

For weeks, I unearthed old journals, cards, words I had forgotten, and pored over it all, caught up in my eight-year-old, fifteen-year-old, and twenty-year-old selves. Moving from journal to journal, cringing at some of what I wrote, I was reminded of who I was back then, and that I wasn't entirely different at nineteen as I was today. Seeing in my small pinched handwriting, "I'm tired," "I'm bored," "I want more," over and over again had me shaking my head, wondering if I should feel bothered or relieved that I continued to feel this way. Books of poetry, letters that I had written but never sent proved I had always been a lover of words. I indulged in them.

In the red shoe box, among cards with get-well wishes and aged brittle roses, was an envelope with *Heidi* written across it in my mom's handwriting. I opened it eagerly like I was unlocking a secret.

There were a few cards from stores I had been to, a business card I didn't recognize, and a coffee card with a few cups punched out on my way to a free cup of coffee. Resting between the cards was a five dollar bill. I noticed the edges were brown, framed by fire, perfectly preserved. My hands shook as I held it by its burnt edges, marveling that it had come this far.

My mom handed me that five dollar bill as I flew down the stairs and out the door eleven years ago. These things were tucked in my wallet, in my purse, in my car as I headed toward a destination I didn't think possible, something childhood dreams are not made of.

I placed the red shoe box beside me on the floor, against my leg, careful not to disturb its contents, as if somehow I could jiggle and disrupt my past by doing so. I noticed a familiar book in the box. It was Scott's favorite childhood book, *The Magical Drawings of Moonie B Finch.* I flipped through the pages and noticed that between pages five and six were folded pieces of paper. I smoothed out the pages, ran my fingertips along the creases, and saw they were letters addressed to me, written by Scott.

I kept still, my breathing shallow, as I remembered.

June 26, 1998

I know we're going to have some tough times adjusting to all of this, but I know we're going to get through it all. I love you, Heidi, and I don't care what you can or can't do. I don't care what you used to be like, or how you are now. I just love you, and I want to be with you. I need you. I need to hear that you love me, too.

Today you opened your eyes and, for the first time, you were in them. Your spirit was in your eyes. It was like hearing from a friend that had gone away for a long time and for a long time you hear nothing. Then one night you get a phone call and they just say, "Hi," but it's the best "Hi" you've ever heard. You were more beautiful in this moment than any other.

He began writing the letters the night after the car crash. Scott and I had been dating a very short time, only six weeks, when time was divided into Before and After. It felt as though a hush fell over the house, over me, as I read the final two paragraphs of the last letter he wrote, the day I came out of my coma.

1
"Do You Want To Live?"

I blinked, my eyes blurred by tears and bright light.

Mom and dad were near, soothing me, but I couldn't understand what they were saying. I knew something had happened. Something bad. But I couldn't remember. I didn't know. My face hot and stretched tight, the tears kept coming. I heard a door open and close.

"Heidi."

My cries turned to sobs.

"Heidi."

I can't stop.

"You were in a car accident. It's bad, Heidi."

It's Scott.

"You've got to fight. Do you want to live?"

Live or die, live or die. I knew it would be easy to die. I was close to it. My parents, Scott, the sterile room, my tears told me death wasn't far.

I answered, "Yes."

I slipped into unconsciousness.

~~~

Pain bled into my dreams, having its way with me. Held captive in cages, I traveled great distances over mountains and through valleys. Hitched to wagons, in truck beds, I bumped over rough terrain and climbed steep hillsides. I was always on my back, unable to curl up or turn to my side; my body stretched out, palms up, and tied down. No time to stop. I slept, but never rested. Sometimes forgotten outside in the cold, I saw my breath and wished someone would take pity on me and bring me inside. There were people everywhere, but I couldn't reach them and they couldn't see me.

Reality crept in once in a while, life and dream crossing lines, blurring together.

A young girl kneeling down, touching my hand, whispering, "We're praying for you. Please be okay." Radio stations being switched and the sound of static. A song I'd recognize, a gentle warning, "Heidi, we're going to pull this out now," as a tube was pulled out of my throat, my body arching and then sighing. Desperate prayers uttered, familiar voices singing to me. These moments formed lullabies breaking through my medicated terror.

Unable to move, my dreams held me under. Throughout my childhood, I was plagued by nightmares, and I learned the art of escaping when I found myself in one. I opened my eyes and shook off the night. But this time, I was trapped in whatever hell my body was in, and my mind refused to let me go.

~~~

Scott returned. "Heidi. You've been in a car accident. Do you know where you are? You're in the hospital. Your right leg is gone. They're trying to save the left one, but it doesn't look good. Heidi? You've been badly burnt. Betty's gone. Heidi?"

My name was a question with no answer. My boyfriend, Scott, was the messenger, and he was forced to repeat this news until I understood, as if I could ever understand. I was told later that morphine made my memory hazy, and I had trouble retaining information. I believe I rejected my messenger's words. They couldn't belong to me.

The extent of my injuries came to me in pieces, in a fog. I saw the wounds on my abdomen first. My skin was red, angry, and gaping. I had smooth skin, a little tanned. It was June, and I had been spending time at the lake.

Why is there a bag over my belly button? Why am I so stiff?

I couldn't move my right arm.

There was so much white—white rolled around my arms, white sheets draped over me, white walls.

I lifted my hand to my face. Something hard and plastic hung from my nose. I tugged on it and gagged. I reached around to my neck, my fingers traveling up, up behind my ears until I felt bandage and skin where my hair should be. Machines surrounded me, pinning me to the bed. They were alive, whirring and flashing, bags of fluid hanging from them. My sight was blurred, fuzzy. I needed my glasses. My hands slid from my bald head and felt long thin tubes attached to my neck near my collarbone.

There was a dull ache at the back of my mind—a memory struggling to free itself.

Car.

Fire.

Betty.

Betty?

Fire.

My legs.

The words flashed through my brain, devoid of images. I didn't remember how, or why, or when it happened, only that I was here, in a hospital, and these words had been given to me, offered up as explanation. I let the words slip through me—one after the other—each word grappling to land, to fit. But, they never found a home.

2

New Life

Scott's mouth moved, buzzed. *This is important, something I should hear.*

"You've been in a drug-induced coma in ICU for two weeks. The doctors thought it was the best thing. They could work on you as often as they needed to. It gave your mind protection and your body a chance to recover."

I tried to nod, but it hurt. Everything hurt.

"You've been moved to the burn unit."

Burn unit?

"You had a punctured lung due to broken ribs…" He gave me a run-down of my injuries. A long list of what had gone wrong. "Burns to over half of your body…Suffering from smoke inhalation…Blood transfusions…Infection…Colostomy bag…Right leg amputated…don't know if the left one can be saved."

Hold on. What? Focus.

"We were worried you wouldn't make it." His voice was calm and even, which I'm sure was an effort.

I made it. Did it matter? The list is so long.

I whispered, "I'm here." I closed my eyes. *No more. No more.*

When my messenger's words sunk in, I gradually became aware that my injuries were serious and devastating. It was a sentence handed to me, and I didn't know what I had done to make me guilty.

I had never broken anything. Not even so much as a sprained ankle. Only a few weeks earlier, I had been grumbling about my foot bothering me when I ran. I went to a walk-in clinic to get to the bottom of the problem. Running was something I did regularly. I loved the rhythm of it and how my mind kept pace with my feet. I learned I had plantar fasciitis, and was told to wait it out. It might go away on its own.

Rest and waiting it out weren't going to heal me now.

My parents didn't have the luxury of a choice when it came time to have my right leg amputated. They signed off in submission to the doctor's decision, a necessity to save me. My leg was a liability, and so it had to go.

Fire had snaked its way to my feet and legs, blazing through muscle to bone, as I hung upside down in my car, suspended by my seat belt. The vinyl seats melted in my red 1988 Nissan Sentra, a car I'd had since I was seventeen. Stringy and sticky, it adhered to my skin, melting me. Fire crept and crawled until it covered 52% of my body. That was the statistic I was given. Just over half of my body burnt. What percent would be erased completely, I wondered. 13%, 18% of a body I could no longer lay claim to.

The crash had taken Betty, my beautiful dark-haired, freckled friend. Betty was gone. Numb, the words zig-zagged through my mind. *Betty is gone, Betty is gone.* She died on impact. These words joined the others. *Betty is gone. She died on impact.*

Betty's earnestness was gone. The way she looked at me when I talked, like I was the only person who mattered. Her smile, her laugh. Gone.

~~~

Scott filled me in on what happened the night of the crash. It was the responsibility of a trauma surgeon at Vancouver General Hospital to fill my family in on the course of action they were taking.

He spoke to my dad, Theodor Kroeker, and Scott. "Heidi has sustained incredible trauma to her body. The back of her body has been burned from her shoulder blades down and the front from her lower abdomen down."

They were prepared to hear this. The doctor in our hometown's hospital had warned them before I was transferred by ambulance to VGH.

"The swelling in Heidi's legs was so severe that we were afraid it was cutting off her circulation, so we cut into her legs to relieve the pressure. What we discovered is her left leg is severely damaged, but may still be useful. However, her lower right leg is damaged beyond repair."

He stopped speaking to both my dad and Scott, and turned all his attention to my dad. "We believe it is necessary to remove Heidi's right foot and part of her leg below the knee, in order to give her a chance. And we need your permission to perform the surgery."

My dad sighed deeply. He squeezed his hands together as his eyes roamed around the room. His heavy German accent broke the silence, "Are there any other tests you can do? Maybe there is something that can be done."

The doctor was compassionate, "Mr. Kroeker, forgive me for being blunt, but Heidi's right leg is literally cooked like a piece of meat. There is nothing that can be done to save it. If we don't remove it, it will kill her." After a moment, the doctor looked down at his clipboard to give him the space he needed.

My dad turned to Scott, "What do you think?" The doctor's gaze followed.

Scott responded, "If it's like he says, I can't imagine anything else that can be done. He's the doctor. If it were my decision, I would let him do whatever he thinks he should do to save her life."

My dad thought for several more seconds. "Ok," his focus returning to the doctor, "please do whatever you can to save her."

"We are, Mr. Kroeker. We're doing everything we can."

I was unconscious as a shaky signature sealed the inevitable, unconscious as surgeons forced their way though muscle and bone to set my new life in motion.

3

Survival

I braced myself. It was morning, nearly seven o'clock.

The small army of the gloved and gowned was about to march into my room. Their accompanying smell of antibacterial soap and the snap of latex gloves was the precursor to sheer agony.

The threat of death was pushed back, and it was time for damage control. Dressing changes were done each morning with the help of strength offered by many hands. I lay on a thick white pad that began at my shoulders, making me look like I had sprouted wings, and stopped at the end of my spine. White gauze surrounded my arms, the remainder of my legs, and my torso; only leaving room for a colostomy bag that sat smack dab in the middle of my abdomen. The thick plastic bag attached to a large pancake-sized beige sticker that lay against me and a stoma, an opening in my body, constructed to collect, well, poop. There was so much damage done by fire, so much grafting, that it was the best solution. I was told it would be temporary. A temporary poop bag.

The pad and gauze were slathered in medicinal ointments the consistency of butter. The ointments dried through the day and night, which affixed the gauze to my skin. Debridement was the term used when nurses ripped the material off, taking healing skin with it. You tear away old skin to make way for new skin.

They could do it slowly or quickly. It didn't matter. Either way, I was in pain. It wasn't like ripping off a band-aid. I wasn't a little girl with a scrape on my knee, my mom crouching, soothing me with promises of, "It's just a quick tear, and it only hurts for a second." No, it wasn't like that at all.

My body was open, raw, and about to receive pain. I wanted to flee, to run. My stomach clenched, and I felt the bile rising in my throat. I thought about people who walked on hot coals, who sought out and welcomed this act of overcoming, like there's nothing you can't do once you've walked on fire. I wondered what they would do if they were in my position, in my bed, living in this near-corpse. They had the luxury of choice, to bear their chosen burden for a few seconds and finish it at will. Would the smell of blood and burnt flesh haunt them? If pieces of them were missing, would they feel like a hero? When my skin was ripped from me each day, I didn't reach a divine place; I couldn't find another entrance to my soul. I was in the dark, torn again and again to create a new body. Not a better body, but a shell that was barely enough.

I'd heard when pain only touches the body, it doesn't interfere with your soul—that time would numb the agony and I would soon forget. What I'd heard was wrong. Suffering sears the soul, and it shreds into a million pieces, just as if I was on fire all over again.

The nurses spoke behind their masks, "Okay, hon, you know what to do. You're going to need to breathe through this."

My body was rigid. My teeth clamped down on the insides of my cheeks.

Rip. Pull.

Lightning quick, pain struck.

I want to scream.

"Breathe, Heidi."

I can't.

Fists clenched, tears rolling down my cheeks, the nurses turned me.

The anticipation of what was coming rivaled the tearing, but I never shut my eyes. I had to see hands land on my body. I had to see the blood-stained gauze.

Rip. Pull.

"In and out. Breathe, sweetie."

I gave in. My breath escaped in short, sharp bursts.

Rip. Pull. Rip. Pull.

This is how I came to love morphine.

In addition to the steady stream of morphine I received, there was a red button on a narrow gray handle I could push to top me up at six minute intervals. It was my very own magic button. It didn't eliminate the pain, but it took the edge off, a faint beep letting me know help was on the way. Inside torture, I clung to control with my left hand. I was a child gripping my security blanket, tethered to the Great Morphine Machine with its promise of comfort and steadfastness.

After debridement, a new back pad was settled into place and fresh gauze wound around me. The nurses turned and adjusted me until I felt comfortable. Comfortable was a relative word here, a fast and loose word I couldn't put any stock into. It was not a simple task. *I* was not a simple task. I often wondered if they dreaded coming into my room, drawing straws to see who got me today. I felt like Humpty Dumpty, cracked open, and everybody scrambling to make the pieces fit. The nurses were gentle and kind, always encouraging, but I'm sure they had to suck in their breath as much as I had to suck in mine whenever they opened my door.

Dr. Brown, the resident doctor, and his students were next. They made their rounds at the burns and plastics unit, checking in with each of their patients. I was in Room 1, the isolation room. I was moved there after being in ICU, and was usually seen last. Sometimes I wielded my patient seniority, having been here for two months, and requested they see me first, so I could speed up the humiliation of seven pairs of eyes of seven strangers seeing me naked and hardly at my best.

Every day, it was the same question. "How are you doing today, Heidi? What's your pain like on a scale of 1 to 10?"

I gave it a beat of thought, pausing to scratch the tip of my nose (morphine made my nose itch), before I measured my pain and answered. "I'm about a 7." It was my standard answer. Not too high, but high enough. I was in considerable pain, even with my friend, morphine. Desperate for relief, my thumb was on that magic button again and again. The pain wasn't as sharp and all-encompassing then, but it never disappeared. It just lay low until the next surgery, the next dressing change, when it jumped high and fast through my body. Pain and I weren't going to be separated anytime soon. 10, 8, 7...did it matter? Pain was everywhere all the time.

I used 7 because I didn't know how I felt anymore. I stuck with 7 because I was resigned to pain. *This is how it is.* If I was lucky enough to be near *okay*, I dropped my number to a 4 or a 5. Those were good days.

Sometimes they didn't believe me. "Heidi, if you're in a lot of pain you need to let us know. We're here to help."

There were times my pain shot sky-high and pain was all I could see. "10. It's a 10 today." Since I rarely used the 10, I was taken seriously.

I was inspected and prodded, checked off and whispered about. I only spoke if I had a question. I tuned them out and willed them away, staring longingly at my TV. The doctors and students were good to me, doing their job, but I was still reeling from the small army of nurses, while trying to catch my breath. Blinding, exploding pain required all of my energy, and being discussed and dissected made me feel like a science experiment. Even though my injuries and the precarious skin grafts required close attention, I couldn't help but feel exhausted, dehumanized, and naked.

When I was given showers while anesthetized, the nurses strategically placed cloths over me as they washed me. I laughed when my nurse, Kathleen, relayed a conversation she had with a doctor. He was puzzled as to why they were doing this. Her response was defensive saying, "Heidi is very modest. We're trying to give her some dignity."

Personal space was a luxury one didn't have at a hospital and I gave in to the fact that I would be seen without a stitch of clothing on regularly, and sacrificed dignity for health. I was a patient, therefore I was defenseless. Removed of my clothes and skin, I had no armor. Cerebrally, I knew the staff was here to heal me, so I contributed by staying still, remaining polite, and being a good girl. I needed them. However, I loathed being the freak show on the table, and my only defense was to turn off my brain, to become numb to my surroundings. The more dependent I was, the less human I felt, and I found a space inside my soul where I clung to choice, even if the choice was to *not* feel.

Once everyone filed out and I wasn't slotted in for surgery, I filled my day with distraction.

Friends and family brought me books, but I was too weak to hold one, and too fragile to read some of what was sent my way. I supposed Christian literature and Christian fiction were meant to cheer me up, but I couldn't take happy endings and girls with heavy hearts, weighing their options only to always come to the right decision after seeking the Lord, and having their problems simply slide off their shoulders as soon as they gave them up to Jesus.

Verses declaring I should "Trust in the Lord for He is the Most High!" didn't interest me. It was brought as provision for my soul with the best of intentions. Ply me with verses and meditations until it would fill in the wound, fill it up and fill it in, until the wound didn't exist anymore. "Let go and let God." Peace would sustain me.

I wanted to be peaceful, and wished I could be comatose along with it. I counted myself among those who believed, but syrupy spoon-fed Christianity wasn't going to cure what was ailing me. I needed love without an agenda. I needed for people to simply be there, and not try to fix me. This wasn't the time to be concerned about my relationship with God. God and I were fine. I was broken, and I would be broken for a while. If I had enough strength, I would have chucked some of those books across the room.

Instead, I invested in television. I used to be too busy to watch TV, and now I had more time than anyone needed. I hadn't watched *Young and the Restless* since I was a girl with my mom. The characters were still here years later. Victor, Nicky, the Abbotts. I picked up where I left off eight years ago. Nothing had changed in Genoa City. I caught up on *Seinfeld* and *Friends*. I watched a travel show religiously. It was on each morning at ten. I never missed an episode. I traveled to India, Israel, Morocco, Thailand… I stayed in out of the way Bed and Breakfasts, rode gondolas, and "tried" the local food. TV was my solace, my reprieve. I didn't have to think. I avoided anything that made me feel too much. I didn't want sappy or anything emotionally charged. Comedy, travel, and over-the-top soap operas were all I could handle.

Visitors were another distraction, something I sometimes welcomed and, at other times, could have done without. With all the people in and out of my room, I couldn't keep track of the new faces I met. I forgot the names of my doctors, and it seemed someone with an important position introduced themselves to me nearly every day. I wanted to stop meeting people.

The resident psychologist popped into my room from time to time, sitting in a chair against the wall next to the door, ready to talk. It was mandatory that he be there, but I had nothing to say to him. His obligatory questions were met with my obligatory answers until time was up. I'm sure I frustrated him with my non-answers, or perhaps I was pretty typical in my unwillingness to "go there" with him.

In a hurry to shoo him out, my replies to his questions didn't matter to me. I doled them out without thinking. I showed optimism during one of our talks when I said, "Things will work out."

He seemed curious. "What do you mean, 'Things will work out?' "

"They just will. I'll be fine."

I didn't know if it was a knee-jerk reaction from Sunday school lessons, that God was in control and I "shouldn't worry about tomorrow because tomorrow will look after itself," or just my great need to be alone that provoked my response.

I offered him the very thing I hated about the verses and books people gave me. I wrapped myself in faith to deflect his questions. The truth was I didn't know what happened. I didn't know how I wound up here. My life was going along just fine until I was hit by a car. One of my very best friends died, and I was here with so much loss, while tied down to a bed. My heart was going to crack wide open if I allowed it. I was its guardian and I believed in *things will work out*. It's all I had left.

Nearly two months had passed in a blur of unconsciousness and operations, and my goal each day was not to make sense of what happened, or even mourn my losses. My goal was to make it through each hour, each day, each surgery, and reach the other side. I needed to get through. My goal was survival.

4

What Remained

I looked at my left foot as if from a long, dark tunnel. When the nurses came in to change the dressings, they warned me, "Don't look, Heidi. It's better for you if you don't look."

I had to look. I needed to see my foot. *What can I still hold on to and hope for?*

They gingerly unwound the white gauze from my foot to reveal toes that were black and red, red and black. I gritted my teeth, pain bitter on my tongue.

"Heidi, can you wiggle your toes at all? How about your big toe? Try the big toe."

I wiggled my big toe, it barely moved. Pain shot through me in a current so strong, I folded in half. I willed my foot into submission. *Please, please hang on. Don't betray me. You're all I have left.*

I didn't want to know the answer to the question, but I had to ask. "Do you think it has a chance? Do you think it's possible for my foot to heal?"

The air in the room changed, thick with anticipation and dread. I pressed a cool cloth against my forehead. All I could hear was the tick-ticking of the small fan in the corner, straining to circulate air and cool me. I was always, always so hot.

"Heidi, it's possible. But, even if it heals enough, it will never be enough. Your foot will always be damaged. There will always be problems. Sometimes..." She stopped and met my eyes. "Sometimes it's better to have the foot amputated and replace it with a prosthetic one. They've come a long way. Sometimes it's better that way."

I imagined myself with my bad foot, dragging it behind me as I limped my way through doorways, up stairs, onto sidewalks. Then I remembered I had a missing foot. The picture changed. Now I had one prosthetic foot *and* my real damaged foot. The picture vanished. *How would this work?*

As the nurses wrapped my foot, bandaging what remained, I knew the truth. It couldn't be salvaged.

We carried on the charade of saving my left leg until August, two months after the crash. Everyone at the burn unit rooted for my leg. I imagined the staff saying, *one leg at a time. She's lost her right. Let's give her more time. She's twenty-three. She's young. She runs. She's young.* Like it was too much for all of us to take in. I could do without one, but not both. Not the left leg, too.

There was a soft knock on my door, and Dr. Brown appeared. He didn't usually come alone, or in the middle of the day. I searched his face for clues, of good news or bad news. I couldn't read him, but if it was good news, he should be smiling. His face was composed, serious.

I held my breath. *Don't say it.*

"We're so sorry."

No, no.

I looked at him.

"We're going to have to take the limb. It's beyond repair."

Take the limb. No.

"I'm sorry, Heidi."

Dr. Brown left, my last chance with him.

The door swung open seconds later, startling me. *What now?* Frozen and wide-eyed, I was a statue of shock.

"Hi, munchkin!" my mom sing-songed. "How are you today?"

"Mom..." I tried again, "Mom. They have to amputate..." I couldn't finish the sentence, the words lodged in my throat.

She rushed to my side, throwing her arms around me. "They were supposed to tell me when they were coming to tell you! They didn't tell me! I was supposed to be here. I'm supposed to be here. Oh, Heidi, it's okay. It's going to be okay."

It wasn't going to be okay. I feared I would never again be okay.

"It's bad enough losing one leg, but both my legs? I will never be the same. What about running? I'll never run. Or hike. Will I be able to hike? Scott and I were going to try rock-climbing this summer." A couple of weeks before the crash, we had gone shopping for new hiking boots for me.

I tried to be positive. "I hear prosthetics have come a long way. Maybe I'll get back into it all again." Every activity, everything I did unfurled in front of me. I didn't know if I could do what I loved again, even with the aid of prosthetic legs.

"I know my foot is bad," I whispered. "I know. I understand they have to take the foot." *The foot.* Already, it didn't belong to me. "Mom, this is really going to happen."

I dug the heels of my hands into my eyes, desperate to hold on in grief. *I knew this was coming. I can't be surprised.* Grief came anyway, pouring down my face and through my fingers. I moved my hands to my lap and watched grief pool in my open hands.

~~~

The day of the surgery, August 10, 1998, I was groggy, sedated in my room to prepare me for the end. Groggy made me more accepting. Railings up on either side, I was imprisoned in my bed as we moved forward, forward to a battle I couldn't win, my leg a traitor.

How much can I lose? When I wake up my foot won't be here. I'll have no feet. Oh my God, why? I don't want this to be my life. Can we just start over?

As I was wheeled to surgery a few nurses stood in the hallway. I tried to smile, to be brave. A nurse spoke, her voice filled with compassion, "Go to sleep now, Heidi. Rest."

5
Cheerfully Noble

"You know you don't have to do this. You know you can go. I'll understand if you can't be here. We haven't been together that long." I whispered to Scott, while machines beeped and clicked around us. We'd only been dating for six weeks when I had my accident.

"I know. Your parents told me the same thing. They were giving me a way out, but I don't want out."

Scott and I met at a church, one we had been attending for less than a year. I had never really spoken to him, even though we traveled in the same circle. I thought he was a little on the skinny side. He was a few inches taller than me with dark hair and light blue eyes. He was quiet and kept to himself.

One evening, we were at an event held at the church and part-way through the evening, he parked himself in the empty chair beside me. As soon as he sat down, I never wanted him to leave. Stillness akin to peace came over me, and I knew it had something to do with him. I didn't know this guy. We had said hello and exchanged a few words. We had friends in common, but I didn't *know* him, and I wanted him to stay.

I found out through a mutual friend that he was interested in me after I had sworn off men at twenty-three, in the rash way that twenty-somethings do by making grand sweeping statements every other week. Even though men were out of my life, he snuck through our friend Nicole's address book to find my phone number.

"He thinks you're smart," Nicole told me. "He likes the way your mind works."

"Really? My mind. He said 'my mind'?" I hadn't told Scott, but that's when he got me—and it forced me to take a deep breath.

My phone rang a week after Nicole played Cupid. It was Scott. "Do you want to go for a walk?"

He showed up at my front door wearing a sweater that I suspected he'd especially worn for me. I hardly knew him, but I figured he wasn't a sweater-wearing sort of guy. It happened to be a warm spring evening, unusual for the lower mainland where April is marked with rain. We walked for a few blocks into town and decided to have a drink at a nearby restaurant. We talked for a while, and I learned he liked to fly planes as well as jump out of them. I learned his eyes were the kind that could see right through you, and when he smiled, it was crooked.

"I'd like to be your friend."

I leaned forward and smiled. "I don't think so. I think you want more than that." I hadn't dated a lot, but past hurts taught me I liked feelings where I could see them, all cards on the table. No pretenses, no bullshit.

He walked me home. We stood at my front door, and I felt light with something new, with the hope of what could be.

We fell hard, fast. Kisses, conversations, and secrets tangled and blurred until we knew this was it, this was love. I saw a future with Scott, but I worried about what that meant. I dated a good friend not that long ago, and it turned out to be a mistake, a grave one. He couldn't accept me. I was too loud, too opinionated, too much. Although he was attracted to me, he thought my personality needed work. He was hopeful. "Maybe you can change." I did. I strove to be fair, quieter, smaller. The relationship was short-lived, and while I was busy becoming less, he extricated himself from us, wanting more.

On high alert, I watched Scott for red flags. I knew I could never be with someone who didn't think I was enough. I waited for Scott to change me. Instead, I found a best friend in my boyfriend. Respectful, funny, and smart, I enjoyed being around him, and I didn't have to defend the walls I built.

Holes were punched in my memory of the week leading to the crash, and my time with him was compressed. *What were all the things we could have done before this happened?*

Scott slid his hand through the railing on my bed and held my hand. "Did I tell you about this weird thing that happened when we first got together?"

"What weird thing?"

"Well, I was sitting on a park bench one day, and out of nowhere these questions ran through my head."

"Okay..."

"What if Heidi went blind? What would you do if she went blind?"

I shivered. "Wow! Really? That *is* eerie. A little foreshadowing. What did you think?"

He had been dating me for such a short while, too short to have thoughts like this enter his mind. He pondered and weighed them because he was that kind of guy. He said, "I thought I'd want to stick around. I'd want to see what you'd do."

Weeks later he received a phone call that echoed the once random questions, which then became otherworldly.

I wondered if we were being prepared for what was coming. My right foot suddenly aching, developing a limp from running; Scott kneeling, gently washing the sand off my feet that rested on a rock at Jericho Beach days before the crash; Scott holding up the camera at the beach while I, tanned in short shorts, squirmed at my photo being taken, that photo later framed and placed bedside at the hospital; Scott and I getting serious fast; calling my friend Angela hours before the crash telling her something felt very wrong, that I was jumpy and anxious, and I couldn't put my finger on it.

We were defensive about what was coming, although there was nothing we could have done. It was unseen and coming at lightning speed. We were tensing, catching our breath, and bracing for impact.

My room was an altar of well-wishes and get-well-soons! all dedicated to me. Heidi "Cheerfully Noble" spelled out and framed in a happy loopy font. Flowers weren't allowed in the burn unit, so teddy bears were brought. Cards were sent and tacked on to the wall. Photographs of me that had been taken before the crash were among the well-wishes. They hung to the left of me, and I found my head turning to them again and again. *It's like I'm dead.*

I stared at the photo of me sitting on the rock, with bare feet and ocean stretched out behind me. I looked so solemn. I knew what I was thinking, *hurry up and take the damn picture already!* It wasn't my face that captivated me, though. It was my legs, my feet. They filled up the photo until they obliterated everything else. I didn't know it would be the last time I would feel my feet scrape against rock, feel gritty sand in between my toes, and know the smooth, taut skin of my legs.

Next to that was a photo of Angela and me on her birthday at a bar downtown. She's sitting on my lap, her arm around me, and I'm posing for the camera, being silly by pressing a fork to my tongue. We're laughing. We were friends before we were roommates, and that photo was up on our fridge for the year we lived together.

My heart slid and sank. *Who am I now?* I was familiar with the smiling, laughing girl, but I didn't know this girl in the bed. I didn't know whether to take her off the wall, or accept that she was still here with me. I didn't know where either of us fit. I wanted to shout to anyone who came through the door, "Take her down! She doesn't belong here."

If it's the shell that's been broken, the temple ruined, could the girl underneath still exist? Would I remain intact, or would you peel back the body and find the insides just as damaged? My body, as I knew it, died that day. *Did I die that day, too?*

I looked at Scott's and my entwined hands and said, "Are you sure?"

His smile was gentle and warm. "This is exactly where I want to be. With you."

6

"I Love You"

Friends and family migrated from watching over me from the waiting room to my room. Gloved and gowned, they shuffled in, tentative and smiling. I smiled in return, seeing they needed reassurance. *Come in, come in.* There were people I hadn't seen in years, people I worked with, and people I lived life with.

My brothers, faithful to their sister, visited often. We were close in age, eighteen months apart; me, Ronald, and Ricardo. We were at that age where we were making our own way, but when it counted, we stood by each other.

For some of my visitors, it was the first time seeing me like this, broken and bandaged, tubes everywhere. They wanted to be there, but didn't know what to say. Some pulled up a chair, there for the long haul. Others were silent as we watched TV together, content to simply be. Some stayed away.

My friend, Lily, came at her mom's insistence. She stood outside the door a few times and couldn't find the strength to come inside. When she finally made it past the doorway, she kept her eye on it and visited with efficiency, quick with questions and answers. All done, she was light on her feet, light with her words. "I have to go!" Turning, hurrying to the door, making her escape. Lily and I had been friends for a long time.

I found myself saying, "It's okay" to almost everyone who stood bedside. I'm not sure who I was trying to convince. No one knew what to say. I knew what they were thinking, how they were overcome with inadequacy, how the right words failed them because they didn't exist. I talked over their discomfort, hiding it with a smile and a quick, "I'll be fine." Instead, I'd ask, "How are you?"

Uncomfortable, no one knew how to answer that question. "I'm here to see you. I'm wondering about you. How are *you* doing?"

"But I want to know how you're doing. It's the same for me every day. Not much changes." I didn't have an answer for them.

Normally words filled my head like ripe apples hanging from their branches ready to be plucked. *Which one will I pick?* Now my mind was spongy, mushy, and my memory a sieve. It slipped and stuttered, shying away from anything bad...and there was so much bad. My mind moved at the same speed as my body, crawling alongside it.

A high school friend, Jason, came to see me. I hadn't seen him since he graduated the year before I did. He stood by my bed and cried, wiping his face. "I'm so sorry. This is awful. This shouldn't have happened. Not to you."

He said, "I wonder if you'll remember. Did the doctors tell you there was a chance you could remember? I had a bad accident at work, and I didn't remember right away but, eventually, it all came back to me."

I'd already had my prognosis. "The doctors say there's a pretty good chance I won't remember. With all the medication and the trauma..." I hoped I would never remember that day. *Trapped in a burning car.* I shook my head.

Most of the week leading up to the crash was wiped out. That day was pieced together for me by everyone else, and it was enough. I counted on mercy and medication to do their work.

"I hope you don't remember."

My friend couldn't have known that I needed his tears. Everybody came in strong, breath sucked in, and bodies rigid. To have someone let their emotions go unchecked relieved me. *This is bad. Please, someone. Tell me this is bad.* I was devastated and, for a few seconds, I wasn't alone.

I had love without condition. No one could have more support than I did, but there were days I felt I was on display. I was at the mercy of anyone who came through my doorway. My face ached with the effort of politeness, and I tired easily. For those days when I couldn't bear to see anyone, I faked sleep. I was eight years old again and my parents were poking their heads into my bedroom to make sure I was asleep. This time it was the nurses who gently pushed the door open and whispered, "Heidi?" I lay still and shut my eyes.

As the nurses got to know me, and me them, I stopped faking and tried the truth instead. They pushed the door open and said, "Heidi, there are people here to see you."

I got bold. "What are their names?"

"I don't know."

I volleyed back, "Well, what do they look like?"

The nurse described them.

"No. Not today. Tell them I'm sleeping." I loved my nurses.

Not sleeping, I took hold of the remote and searched for pain management in the form of television. I looked around my room, taking stock, still in shock that I ended up here. The first and last time I spent time in a hospital was as a baby.

I come from a long line of doers. Good Mennonite stock that emigrated from Paraguay, South America. Born in Vancouver, my brothers and I were destined for a North American life. Being a Mennonite meant there is nothing you can't fix by doing. In church circles, it's called the gift of hospitality. It was like a calling for us as Mennonites. You don't sit around and wait for things to fall into your lap. We may be pacifists in war, but in life, you cook, clean, and bake! I had a lot of family who wanted to help. When I was at my worst, no one knowing if I was going to cross over to the other side, family came out in droves. My brothers, aunts, uncles, and cousins parked themselves on chairs in the waiting rooms and took turns sitting with me while I was oblivious to what was going on around me.

One of my cousins was willing to donate skin. Some were silently supportive, stoic in their pacing around the room. Others sat with me and held my hand. Some prayed and recruited their church congregations in prayer. Others had questions for the doctors. *What can we do? How can we help?* This is the Mennonite way. There may be a situation which is beyond our control, but one can always find a way to help. We demonstrate our love through action. The gift of hospitality is never in short supply.

Another way we help is through food. There is always more than enough food. You don't go without, not if my mom or any of her sisters have anything to say about it. I have never left one of our family gatherings without somebody pressing food into my hands saying, "For lunch tomorrow." You look down and it's already been covered in plastic wrap, or tucked into a Tupperware container. You cannot refuse. It's not a choice. You say thank you and go, grateful for how your body will be nourished tomorrow.

I grew up in a house where you pray, but with efficiency. Short and to the point, amen. God doesn't need for you to go on and on. He's a busy God and not interested in flowery prose. He's God. He knows your needs. My prayers growing up were all said in German. They were memorized, traditional prayers— one for mealtime, and one for bedtime.

As a child I believed God preferred German. It was the language I learned first, passed down from my parents and their parents, who were German Russians. If I said a prayer in English, it would not be received as well as if I had spoken it in German. Our prayer at mealtimes went like this, *Segne Vater diese Speise uns zur Kraft und Dir zum Preise. Amen.* (Father, bless this food for our strength and to You as praise) It is said swiftly but with reverence.

To amuse ourselves, my brothers and I recited it as fast as we could, picking up speed as we went along. It was a race. Who could finish first?

"SegneVaterdiesespeiseunzurkraftunddizumprciseamen!"

My dad did not appreciate this. With a stern look and a "Nah" with the 'a' drawn out, so it came out a Naaah, the word coming up at the end, we shut up and looked down at our plates, very busy with our forks. This meant he also didn't appreciate when we said it slowly enunciating each word as if we were delivering a powerful sermon, sometimes with emphatic arm gestures. This was considered disrespectful, too. I'm pretty sure I saw my dad hiding a smile more than once during our attempts to spice up our prayer lives.

My parents were at the hospital almost every day, usually together. Petting, fussing, caring, they were a team, a united front of service. I was surprised to see my dad alone this day, and I put the remote down. He looked like he had something on his mind.

"How are you today, Heidi?"

"I'm okay. Tired."

He stood at the foot of my bed and cleared his throat. He looked down, then up. "When you were brand new to the world, I dedicated you to God. I told Him, she is Yours first, and mine second." He spoke in his well-worn German broken with English, the voice of my childhood.

I looked at his calloused hands, tough from years of cutting wood and cabinet-making. The same hands that cradled me when I was a newborn, carrying me around in the middle of the night to lull me to sleep. From infancy on, I liked to be near him. There's evidence of this in photos of us sitting side by side, my dad sipping his Yerba Mate (a South American herbal tea) and me leaning into him. My brothers and I spent a lot of time on my dad's back as he crawled around on all fours as a bucking bronco, a galloping horse. He wrestled with us, played street hockey with us, but he never said *I love you*. We were loved; it didn't need to be said.

He continued, "I prayed, wondering if God was going to make good on the dedication. But, God gave you back to us." He paused, looked at the floor, and then his eyes met mine. "I love you, Heidi."

7

Standing Guard

Justice was on my mom's mind. With the Abbotsford local paper tucked under her arm, she said, "They're not sure if they're going to charge the driver. Can you believe it? After what he did?"

She usually kept any behind-the-scenes news to herself. Focused on my recovery, she didn't want anything or anyone to get in the way. And I didn't want to know. It took so much energy to be here in this bed that I couldn't think about the driver who started all of this.

"They've been writing about you and Betty in the paper. *And* the driver. We've been talking to the police." She stopped, unsure if she should go on. "This is what a reporter wrote just days after the accident." She handed me the paper and pointed to the article.

"Abbotsford City Police are still investigating to determine if charges will be laid against the 17-year-old driver of the Chevy Malibu involved in Friday's fatal car accident.

Preliminary investigation results show the eastbound Malibu overtook another vehicle shortly before the crash, Constable Elly Sawchuck said. But she said it was too early to tell exactly how fast the car was going and whether it was "drag-racing" the other car at the time of the collision.

"Speed was definitely a factor," she told *The News* yesterday. The driver, who was treated and released from MSA Hospital after the crash, refused to provide a blood sample.

Neighbors, who were among the first on the accident scene, were upset at the peculiar behavior of the Chevy Malibu's two occupants, who they said seemed more concerned with damage to their car than the injuries suffered by the girls.

Ray Brault, who lives nearby and raced to the scene after hearing "a hell of a bang" said the pair were using profanities and criticizing the girls for pulling out in front of them."

My mom was quick to soothe me. "Heidi, I know you. I know how you drive. You wouldn't have left the stop sign if it was unsafe." She smiled, "And your car is too slow."

I closed my eyes and tried to conjure up the memory. "I don't remember anything about the day. Not a thing. What if I thought I could make it?" Hanging between us was, what if it was my fault? What if I was the reason Betty wasn't here?

"The police asked me about that. They wondered if you misjudged the speed they were going, or if you were speeding. But I told them I know my daughter. She's a good driver with no record. She wouldn't have done it. Heidi, you didn't do this. These boys…this boy…they were going too fast."

I knew myself and knew the intersection well. We lived right around the corner from it. I had moved back in with my parents for a while after being on my own, and they had lived there since I was twelve.

"Our neighbor saw you stop at the sign," she said. "He saw you stop," emphasizing that I had followed the rules. "Your dad and I are not going to let them get away with it. People heard them," she lowered her voice, "*swearing* when you were down there…in the car."

I could handle the story in pieces, small pieces. Every time I was given a new piece, it felt like I was being cut and slashed with information. I shook with anger hearing these guys were worried about their car, and actually cursed at us while we were trapped in a car on fire. *Who does that?* I could understand shock. I grasped fear. But I could not comprehend indifference, and I could not fathom cruelty. I didn't want to be angry. I didn't want to waste energy thinking about them, speculating about their feelings. I had to concentrate on getting better, and I couldn't let them in. It was too much. It was all too much.

"Let's talk about something else, Mom. I'm tired."

She patted my hand. "You're right." She drew her shoulders back. "Can I get you anything?"

"I'd love some juice."

"Okay. Orange?" she smiled, happy to be needed.

On my own again, I mulled over the staff's concern of my isolation mentioned earlier that day. They thought it could improve my health to share a room with another patient—it would be good for us to "talk it out." I hoped that time would never arrive. Since childhood, I worked through problems alone, and prided myself on my independence and self-sufficiency. My brothers and I were great playmates, but I loved being the eldest, the only girl, and how much time I was given on my own. I asked advice of friends and processed aloud, but when it got to deep-down soul-searching, I preferred doing it alone. I couldn't imagine having to make small talk with a stranger who slept next to me.

Everyone who came to visit was mourning, and anyone staying at the hospital was mourning. Sharing a room with another patient would be multiplying grief, and I didn't know if I could handle more. I managed grief all of the time, juggling it from one side of my brain to the other. When I was alone or asleep, I didn't have to manage it as much, think about it as much. And I wasn't really alone. I had family, Scott, and my best friends.

The life and loss of Betty was between Angela, Loraleigh, and me. Betty had introduced me to Loraleigh. I had introduced Betty to Angela. We were linked by this sharing of each other, sure in the knowledge of you-will-love-her as soon as you meet her. We did. We loved each other within minutes of meeting the other.

Angela and I were introduced to each other when we were eighteen through my friend and her boyfriend at the time. He was convinced we would like each other. Angela and I became friends and then roommates for a year when we were 21. I moved back home afterward to save some money and plan for the future, contemplating returning to school, maybe becoming a teacher.

Angela was studying to be a nurse and during quieter times, she'd sit at the edge of my bed and share the far-reaching effects of what had happened.

She had arrived at the hospital moments after Betty and I were brought into emergency at our local hospital. She was at work, waitressing, when her friend, Mark, told her she needed to come with him, that something had happened. She followed, untying her apron, icy fear trickling down her spine. She left her tables, her customers, and handed her money to the hostess. In his car, on the way to the hospital, he explained. He lived nearby and happened to be home when the cars collided. He discovered who had been pried out of the red car and, as smoke billowed and police officers closed the road, he knew he needed to get Angela. "Heidi's in emergency. It looks like her legs…"

She gasped, "Did she break her leg?"

Mark answered, "No. It's worse than that. This is bad, Ang."

The icy fear returned to her spine. She whispered, "Betty?" Angela knew we had been on our way to her restaurant.

He shook his head.

When Angela finally went home that night, she listened to the messages waiting for her on the answering machine. Betty greeted her, "Thought I could catch you before you left. We're on our way to see you!" Bubbly, happy Betty.

Angela touched my hand. "If only I was home to answer her call. I could have delayed her, even if just by seconds. Those seconds haunt me."

I looked at my friend. She didn't have to tell me how alone she felt, losing one friend to death and another to the hospital.

Her eyes gave away her loneliness. I whispered, "There was nothing you could have done. Don't do that to yourself."

A small smile crossed her face, "I can't erase her voice from the machine. I won't let my roommates touch it. I miss her."

"Me too. I miss her laugh."

We were silent for a moment before I asked what had been on my mind. "Can I tell you something and you won't judge me or think I'm weird?"

Many of our conversations began with my request for no judgment, so she indulged me. "Go for it."

"I had this moment a while ago where I could just feel her, like she was in the room with me. And I think she's in a good place, like she was home. I think she's okay, Ang. I could see her smile and hear her voice. I thought I heard *it's beautiful here*. Is that crazy?"

Tears shone in Angela's eyes. "No, not crazy at all."

We were silent for a moment, our unshed tears between us.

Angela filled in the gaps of time between the crash and coma. "We weren't sure that you'd make it. More than once we were told to say our goodbyes to you. And then you'd come around. I got to know Scott. We spent all this time together. Bonding over grief," she laughed. "He's solid, Heidi. A good guy."

It was my turn to smile, "I'm glad you like him. It's important to me that you like him."

Drugs and surgery created a gulf between my body and my emotions. When Angela visited, she became a mirror for my anguish, naming what I couldn't explore. She was one of the few people I could talk to. I found solace in her friendship, in our shared loss.

Loraleigh flew from Winnipeg days after the crash and stood vigil by keeping a journal through the month of June into the first few days of July.

June 18, '98
"The doctors and nurses all keep saying that your life will never be the same again. I believe it, but I think I believe it in a different way than they do."

June 24, '98

"Tuesday we talked to the doctor. He had some good news, but always along with good news comes the bad news. The good news was that they're going to take the tube out of your mouth soon and slowly let you wake up. That will be good. I hope they brush your teeth for you. I'm sure you'll feel like your teeth have about fifty billion sweaters over them! The bad news is that the infection in your leg is getting worse and there is talk of amputating further, above the knee. I don't want that for you. I didn't want them to shave your head, either, but they did. In some ways, I feel a little responsible for all your changes. We watch the doctors do all this to you, and it kills me that they don't even ask you what you want. I want to ask you but it's not that easy right now."

June 25, '98

"Oh, Heidi!" Wow, what a treat to see you today! It's a treat to see you every day but what a treat to see you today. Your eyes are open and you even squeezed my hand! Sometimes I think those little things are more for us than for you. I even got a smile! Heidi, I'm just so happy for you."

I loved reading her words, her heart splayed on the pages. My mom and my friends shouldered sorrow together. While I fought for my life, they stood guard, tending to me with grace and dignity. When I couldn't fight, they fought on my behalf, defining love.

8

Pain Management

I was in Room 1, specially equipped for my survival. It was an isolation room to protect me from others, and to protect others from me by keeping infection out.

Room 1 meant hands must be washed upon entering and leaving the room. It meant not only nurses, but visitors must also don masks, gloves and gowns to see me. A central line carried my medicine that hung in clear full bags. The empty bags shriveled until they were dry, then were swapped for another full bag. A tube inserted into my stomach through my nose fed me a thick putty-colored liquid containing my daily nutrients. There was also a tube inserted into my urethra to drain it, morphine to manage pain, and a steady supply of oxygen.

My nurses were my primary caregivers and my guides to survival.

Joan was called upon to position me in the bed to get me comfortable if no one else could. She had a knack. Marion missed nothing, including my attachment to the travel program, and made sure the TV was flicked on to the right channel, hurrying the dressing changes along to accommodate me. When she returned from her trip to Turkey, she brought me a miniature Turkish rug and tacked it onto the wall. "For your future travels," she said.

Kathleen's anecdotes about her life bordered on over-sharing, and I adored her. She spent time with me and was my anchor to the outside. Ann answered my questions, and if she didn't know, she never pretended otherwise, no platitudes. When the mood was somber, Kelly had an uninhibited laugh that cut through the dark. Julie was small and quick, her curly hair bouncing as she moved from task to task. She said, "One day you'll visit, and I won't recognize you. I've told other patients who come back to 'pull your hair back and get on the floor!'" She laughed, "I have a hard time recognizing former patients because they come in upright."

My room was a revolving door of nurses, and over time they became family.

My nurses manifested healing. Their sure, deft hands were the perfect balm to my devastation. It was how they told me funny stories about their families and pinned get-well cards to the wall. It was the warm blankets they tucked me into, and the banana milkshakes they made to fatten me up. It was the conversations we had.

The Head Nurse, Carol, spoke to me about the week that involved scheduling an upcoming shower.

I interrupted, "I can't believe I'm a burn victim. I used to put money in the boots of the firefighters who stood outside grocery stores and malls collecting money for people like me. I'm that person."

"We don't use the word victim here," she said. "You're a survivor. Don't forget that."

Survivor. "Oh." I said it out loud. "Survivor. Right. I guess that's what I'll be."

"That's who you are."

We resumed our discussion of the impending shower. They were given once a week. It's a burn shower, which meant I was placed on a stainless steel gurney and wheeled to a large sterile room where spigots hung from the ceiling, ready with a plan and purpose. These showers were excruciatingly painful. I had always viewed water as cleansing, healing. Here, it was the enemy, pointed and sharp as it sliced through my many open wounds and grafts that were healing. Thankfully, I was given a drug called Ketamine.

Ketamine is a fast acting anesthetic and painkiller and is known for its dissociative properties, and can make a person feel a sense of detachment, as if their mind is separated from their body. Its primary use is in veterinary surgery, but it's also sold illegally, used recreationally, and slipped into drinks, gaining its moniker as the date rape drug.

Just before the shower, the anesthesiologist administered the drug, and I drifted off. I was usually given enough of this drug to knock me out.

I can hear them. My doctor, my nurses. They're discussing my central line, the IV that feeds into me.

"She needs a new one. We'll take out this one and put in a new line."

I can hear him. My doctor.

And feel their hands.

This isn't supposed to happen. I know this. I try to blink, to open my eyes. I can't.

I can't distinguish the nurses' voices. I know there's more than one. There's always more than one, but somehow they have merged into one voice, one nurse.

I can't move, I can't move. My eyes won't open. Focus, focus.

I will my hands to move, just a flutter, to signal I'm here. I don't know if anything's happening. Can they see my hand?

Short of breath, my heart is racing. I'm choking on fear.

I can't move! I can hear my doctor. There is no pain, but I can feel the nurse's hands.

I'm awake.

"Her pulse is climbing."

"She needs oxygen."

"What's going on?"

"Give her oxygen."

I want to speak, to open my mouth.

Please.

When I fully awoke, I realized that what had taken place wasn't a dream or a gone-sideways morphine trip. Carol was the first person I saw afterward. "I was awake during the shower and paralyzed. I could hear talking, but I couldn't do anything."

Carol was calm, "No harm was done to you while you were under the anesthesia. This is one of the possible side-effects of

Ketamine. Do you know you've sung during a shower before, giddy and oblivious to what was going on? Don't worry, Heidi. We'll do everything we can to prevent it from happening again."

If it happened with Ketamine, though, could it happen with another anesthetic? I was worried about waking up during surgery. Worried about being cheated and feeling pain. Worried about being frozen, and no one knowing.

I gave voice to my fear, "I was so scared. You'll do everything you can?" aiming for nonchalance but looking for reassurance.

Carol could see right through me. "Trust me."

~~~

I often didn't know the time. Keeping time didn't mean anything to me until the morning broke. I was alerted to the day's lateness when lights dimmed and people spoke in hushed voices, and visitors had long since gone. I was alone. All nights were the same here. I just hunkered down anticipating the next morning's rigorous routine.

On this particular night, it was quiet, too quiet, and all of the thoughts I tried desperately to avoid all day came pouring in. I thought of my visitors who came to see me, how I envied their ability to leave. They could exit the hospital and resume their lives. *I can't escape. I can't ditch this for an afternoon.* They could shed the claustrophobia of my room, of what my life had become, and walk on healthy legs supported by strong bodies. *Life goes on, but not for me.*

Some nights I could distract myself by watching enough TV that my head was full of witty quips and sarcastic banter, which would lull me to sleep. But not that night. That night I lay on my bed wondering how in the hell I ended up here, the weight of the surgeries, the finality of my losses totaling up and streaming down my face.

Kate, my nurse that night, came in to check on me. She checked my vitals and strapped the blood pressure cuff to me. As the cuff tightened around my arm she reached for my hand, held it until my tears subsided. "Is there anything I can do?"

"No."

Her quiet acceptance was enough.

I woke up to loss and went to bed with it. I aged overnight. Pieces of me were missing and the rest was red and raw, hurting and oozing. I didn't have legs that stretched all the way out to the end of the bed, toes wiggling and feet ice cold. Consumed with how they weren't there anymore, I wildly thought, *maybe they could be!* I'd heard of miracles like this in far-off places, in remote villages in Africa. You never heard stories like this happening in the town next to you. Maybe I could be that story. Maybe my legs would lengthen, grow, if I believed enough. These thoughts were quickly reigned in and stamped out, sanity winning. My heart was another matter, and wasn't so easily tamed. It wanted more.

I was often asked, "Weren't you, aren't you angry?" Anger wasn't what fueled me to keep going. It wasn't that I didn't get angry, but anger wasn't what woke me up and provoked me. Hard to explain and difficult to define just what it was that I said yes to each day, except there was a hanging-on, a white-knuckled grip on my life that this couldn't be it. My life would not end in this bed, my body present but vacant, summed up by what I'd lost.

I didn't want to be beaten. I longed to get better. Hope staved off the emptiness, like fog rolling in when it came, propelled by loss, seeking to hold me in its jaws. I refused to settle for an existence. I was after life.

9

A Girl Again

Skin, our largest organ, there to protect us, was failing me. The surgeons were doing damage control, but the damage was always a step ahead of them, gaining and unstoppable.

A staph infection called MRSA (Methicillin-Resistant Staphylococcus Aureus) made its rounds in the hospital, and it was only a matter of time before I was its next target. I was an easy one. I had open wounds, a compromised immune system, which is the perfect candidate for this super bug. Anyone could have given it to me. It can live on door handles, floors, almost any surface. People can carry it and never know. It's resistant to antibiotics, so it's difficult to eliminate. I got infected, and it unleashed havoc with my recovery.

A sign was taped to the outside of my door warning others to proceed with caution. Upon entry, gloves and gowns had to be worn, and hands washed thoroughly to prevent the spread of infection. Being MRSA positive, I was in isolation, and a danger to myself and anyone who touched me.

It was September, three and a half months since the crash, and I was in trouble. MRSA waged war, and my backside wasn't healing because my skin grafts weren't taking. Skin grafts are where two layers of healthy skin, the epidermis and the dermis, are taken from a healthy part of the body, a donor site, and transplanted to the part of the body that needs it. This is all done under general anesthesia. I came to know this as harvesting.

Skin was harvested from my head, my arms, and my back multiple times. Once the fog of anesthesia cleared and I vomited the contents of my stomach until the bile turned green, I felt beaten up, wasted, and my pain was at a 10. When I first heard the word "harvest" in conjunction with my skin, it was all wrong. Harvest normally conjures images of Thanksgiving, farms, leaves of red and gold. Now harvest meant healthy skin shaved off some part of my body and stretched across other parts of my body that were open and vulnerable to infection.

Recovery could be long after harvesting, and it was especially long after being infected with MRSA. Pain was hot and high on my pain scale, so it was hard to find a comfortable position in bed. If my back or bum or arm pressed against the bed, I felt like I was being branded with a hot iron over and over again. The pain would overwhelm all of my senses, so I couldn't eat, rest, or breathe properly. The nurses and orderlies shifted me in small increments, to the left or right, until I felt relief.

One morning Dr. Brown came to see me, "Heidi, how are you?"

I was honest and a little embarrassed. No modesty. "My bum really hurts."

"I know," he said, kindly. "We're going to take care of that. We'll talk soon."

I knew that meant another surgery, and all I could do is wait to be told when.

After each surgery, I looked different. A small mole from my back was transplanted to my leg. The skin from my arm was moved to wrinkle over my rib cage. My skin, stretched and stitched, looked like gingham.

I am a carefully woven patchwork quilt.

My doctors came up with a proposal. "Since your backside isn't healing and you lie on your back and bum all day, every day, let's put you on your stomach for three days at the least, and five days at the most, after the next surgery. We'll put a little extra morphine in your IV to make you more comfortable."

I said yes without hesitation. What choice did I have? This was my best shot. I needed to heal, and my butt was killing me.

The nurses would take on the challenge as well, attempting to make me as comfortable as possible under the unusual circumstances. Lying on my stomach for three, possibly five days, wasn't going to be an easy feat. My army of nurses would be reduced to one or two a day. Doctors and their students wouldn't enter the room. There would be a large dressing, but that would remain untouched. Instead, I'd be left to rest on my stomach over the next few days after surgery. I didn't need to be turned, since I was going to be immobilized. An army wouldn't be needed.

I woke up after a long surgery, on my stomach. My arms were at my sides, positioned for recovery, and a back pad, my white wings, stitched to me. My food pumped and chugged through my nose to my stomach. The Great Morphine Machine seemed to bow to me at my right, sending me blinking messages in red, promising to be steadfast. Morphine clouded my brain and kept me safe. It was dangerous for me to think ahead, to consider the hours stretched out before me. Pain, held at bay, was less alive, blunt and distant. Now I was faced with a different torment. I was trapped with no chance of rescue for days, mummified alive.

I could move my head slightly to the right or left. The nurses fastened a hand mirror to the bed on my right side, a perfect reflection of the TV in it, keeping me in a comedy coma. When my eyes weren't open, canned laughter and outraged gasps filled my head.

The hospital carried an odor of medicine, and disinfectant, sick, and untouched food, and that never changed. I didn't realize weariness had a smell until I got here.

My nurses faithfully topped up my morphine, allowing me to sleep more and leave me in a fog. My pain dulled, I couldn't see much, but my hearing was heightened. I was sensitive to every drip, sigh, and squeak as the nurses tiptoed their way out the door. I heard the swish of their scrubs as the door swung closed. I didn't have many visitors during this time, preferring my TV and morphine, instead. When people came they stayed for seconds, spoke softly, and left, the door swinging shut behind them. *Swish.* Taking off their gowns and gloves. *Slide, snap.* I needed to conserve my energy for the marathon.

Three days dragged by. My mom and Scott came to see me. We exchanged few words, and they only stayed to check in, to ask if I was okay, and to encourage me to hang on. *You're doing great.* They were a reminder of this burden and how long I'd been here. If they stayed too long, I was afraid I'd panic. I had carefully constructed my mental walls, and they could not crumble. Everything I had, and there wasn't much of me left, focused on preservation. I didn't want to talk. Words cost, and speaking an extravagance I couldn't afford. It was best to be isolated.

The doctors communicated through the nurses. "How are you? Do you think you can handle more? Maybe one or two more days? You're doing so well."

Again, I said yes. I had to do this. If my body could mend using sheer will, I would come through this whole, as though my body never caught on fire. I had to make this surgery count.

When awake, I prepared my body for what lay ahead. In my morphine stupor, I believed it would be a great opportunity to work at the thick white pad affixed to me, whose ointments had dried and become loose. I was a contortionist, freeing up my hand to snake its way to my shoulder and pick, pick at the padding.

If I can just reach this shoulder.

I'm itchy.

If I can control one thing.

It is tomb-like in here.

If I tear my skin now, it will hurt less when the army returns.

I hurt myself at my own hands rather than wait for someone else to do the hurting. Everything was done *to* me, and though it was no less painful, exerting my will, gritting my teeth, and causing my own anguish gave me power. Pain, large and violent, was on its way, so if I could do it now at my pace, in no hurry, it lessened the blow.

One of the nurses made her way into the tomb and noticed my handiwork. "You shouldn't be doing this," she said. On her way out, she patted my bare shoulder, the one I had been working on. We were nearing the end of the marathon, the end of my immobilization, and my handiwork wouldn't do too much damage. The door opened and closed. *Swish.* I got to work on the next shoulder.

I stayed on my stomach for five days.

The experiment was a success. The grafts took this time. My body precariously knit together and held. I made it, and I was finally released from my mental coffin.

My fear appeased, I breathed deeply again. *Please, let me never ever have to do that again.* I knew this was one of the hardest things I'd ever accomplish in this room. We won this battle. The doctors were optimistic that we would be ahead from now on, that our side would continue to win the war against MRSA. Since MRSA was still present, the sign remained on my door, and I remained isolated. I was pumped full of antibiotics and my nostrils were swabbed every few weeks, a q-tip pushed high up my nose to test for the superbug. The tests always came back positive and while the doctors and nurses did everything they could to wipe it out, MRSA hung on, living with me for a year.

A week later I lay on my side, propped up by a fortress of pillows. I was still fragile, but recovering. I wrapped my hand around my bandaged upper arm, my fingertips meeting. I had withered away to ninety pounds. It took much energy to be a burn survivor, so keeping weight on proved to be difficult. I looked down at my legs. I preferred them covered up, but today I peeled back the blankets to inspect the wounds on my legs.

The dressings were off to allow for air to reach the open spots. My legs, especially my right, were in bad shape. I had skin that adhered to the bone and my right knee had a deep wound the size of a quarter that was troublesome and seemed determined to stay. I should be fitted for prosthetics soon, but my legs weren't ready.

It was easier to itemize my issues rather than face my feelings.

I poked the red, raw hole in my knee, and glared at it. As it began to throb, loneliness squeezed my chest, surprising me. I expected hatred to surface, but the loss of my skin and legs wrung out my heart. I felt forsaken. There were people right outside my door. With a push of a button I could summon someone to me, but what would I say to them once they got here? I was alone with the ugliness of my injuries, with sadness that threatened to crush me. I pulled the blanket over my legs, over the monstrosity, and jabbed at the button on my remote. I watched the TV flicker to life and forced myself to set aside further feelings of despair.

Things jumped from desperate to relief quickly here, and I ping-ponged from one thing to the next. I was sacrificed to be a patient, feeling lost in procedure and protocol. The hospital was a place where pain became another sense. It was a part of me as much as seeing or hearing. I needed something to hold onto, something to tie me to the young woman who had a future.

I was awake and alive enough now to contemplate what would happen next. Direction existed again, and I wondered where I would go and how would I reach a path, any path, when I was held down by the present. I looked up at the clock on the wall, the seconds ticking by, and wished for a window to show me what lay ahead, to see a place I hoped wouldn't be bare.

A knock at my door interrupted my thoughts. "Heidi, would you like a warm blanket?" It was Denny offering.

If it was possible to have a favorite thing about the hospital, it was warm blankets. When I no longer had to have sheets tented over me to prevent anything from sticking to me, relief was offered in warm blankets. Blankets were put into a blanket warmer, a stainless steel contraption, and retrieved, sterile and warm, smelling clean and clinical. After each surgery and every procedure, a blanket was snapped over me, landing like a sigh.

I welcomed the offer, and he quickly returned with a warm blanket in hand.

Denny was an orderly I adored. Big and burly, he had arms like Popeye. His laugh boomed and bounced off the walls, leading the way, so I knew when he was near. He was there to help, and no task was too big or too menial. He helped the nurses turn me in my bed. He lifted me onto surgery gurneys. He helped wash my face.

Denny tucked the blanket around me while inquiring after my beauty regimens. "Are you looking after your face?" Before I could answer, he said, "If not, let's get started. Women need to look after themselves."

Is he serious? Is he making fun of me? I took a long look at him and decided that he was serious. I hadn't looked into a mirror in months. "I don't have cleanser."

"Well," he said, "we need to fix that."

The first time I looked at myself was through a handheld mirror a nurse held up for me. She had asked, "Are you ready?"

I'd nodded. What was there to be sensitive about? My body bore the brunt of the damage. I was told my face was mostly fine, except for a burn near my chin.

My reflection showed a different story. My shaved head had become a main supplier of healthy skin to the rest of my body. I searched the mirror, taking further inventory. There was an angry-looking wound close to my right temple from a razor that had cut too deep. My cheeks were sucked in, my eyebrows needed tending, and there was a red puffy scar that curved around the right side of my chin.

Tears stung my eyes and I furiously wiped them away. *I don't look like me.*

I stared at my green eyes for a while, the only part of my face that reminded me of myself. They were too large in my hollow face, but I recognized them. I broke the stare when I had enough. *Enough change, enough for today.*

But Denny changed all that. When it was slow and quiet in the evenings, Denny would come into my room and help me wash my face.

My mom bought cleanser, cotton pads, toner, and one of those plastic pouches with a bright floral pattern you get at a drugstore to hold it all in. My right arm was weak. No one knew why. I had trouble using it, so Denny was my arm. He sat at the edge of my bed, wet a cloth, poured cleanser on it and washed my face.

He patted my face dry and dabbed it with cotton pads doused in toner. "You see?" he grinned, "You need to feel like a girl again."

And slowly, as my face was wiped of each day's routine and tears that had been left unchecked, I breathed in the faint scent of mint, my face squeaky clean, and I felt myself transported to my bathroom at home again, staring in the mirror before I tucked in for the night. Even though my body was ravaged by fire, even though my feet were gone, my eyes were open. I was still me, a girl who needed to take her rightful place in her own body.

I was a girl, and that mattered.

10
The First Step

Time stood still inside the walls of the hospital. It was early October, month five of my stay. While summer gave in to fall, the dull white of the floors, the walls, and the sheets stayed the same. Food trays were dropped off and picked up. Dirty laundry was scooped up and fresh sheets were spread underneath me, rolling me back and forth like dough on a floured tray, until the sheets were tucked and even. Shoes squeaked up and down the scrubbed floors. Nurses went on breaks and returned. I continued to recover and watch TV.

I had lost track of how often I was wheeled in and out of my room, conscious and unconscious, but I knew the number was high, nearing twenty. Fasciotomies, exploratory surgery, amputations, debridements, and grafts, I spent hours and days in the operating room. Surgeries slowed down, and it was time to break the monotony of my days. I was going to meet the prosthetist, my leg guy, as I would later come to call him. I had no idea what would be involved. How long would it take? How did one go about making legs? I hoped I'd be given answers.

Everything here was about waiting. Wait for the next surgery. Wait for the doctor to come see me. Wait to heal. Wait until I'm told what to do next. I couldn't will anything to happen faster. I couldn't make anything go. I was at the mercy of my body. Even my resourceful doctors were following my body's lead. We were all waiting. If one could hone the skill of survival, it was going to be me. I could do very little besides read a chapter of a book or watch television, so survival became my craft, and I was good at it.

Later that day, David, my prosthetist, entered my room to discuss fitting me for prosthetic legs. "Hello, Heidi," he said, running his fingers through his thinning white hair and adjusted his glasses. "It's nice to meet you."

I wasn't sure of the time, but I knew it had to be late, and wondered why it took him so long to get here. To my dismay, I found out it was actually early afternoon. Morphine messed with my days, or maybe it was each day running into the next that messed with keeping track of time.

This discussion of my legs, one of many, was a step forward to getting me closer to my goal, and I was anxious to begin the process. Acquiring legs was the key to getting my life back, to returning to the world I knew. I might not be the same in it, but I ached for normal, and I knew this is what it would take to achieve that. I had to walk.

Cheerfully, David talked about casting me. "Hmmm…this will be interesting." That was the word he used to explain the open wounds on my legs. An *interesting* problem. Would it be worth it to put all of this plaster on me, maybe damaging my skin further? And it would hurt.

But everything hurt. I had become hyper-sensitive. Even running water on my skin caused me pain. It was like my body had enough, and my nerve endings became live wires. I had been in the burn unit for months, and my body needed space, always crying out for it to be left alone.

I couldn't imagine how he did his job of dealing with people with missing limbs, meeting them in trauma and having to maneuver each situation so carefully. I may have been one out of a hundred, but he was still tactful, still sensitive. This wasn't new for him, but this was completely new for me. With care and forthrightness, he explained how the process worked.

His fingers rested on his chin as he offered up a smile. "Well, I've got some problem solving to do. I'll be back soon. And then I'll cast you."

I saw David about a week later. He handed me a pair of thick squishy liners that looked like super-sized rubbery socks, or giant condoms. They were comical, especially when they bent in half when I held them. "You're going to roll those over your legs. Well, not this time. Gail and I will help you with that."

I didn't have the strength, yet. I could barely bend my body far enough to reach my legs. David would get help from the burn unit's resident physiotherapist, Gail. Since my legs were in various stages of healing and some parts were still open and fragile, she dusted powder on my legs to make it easier to slip the liners over my legs and create a barrier. She stretched and pulled until they were over my legs.

He spread plaster over the liners and waited until it hardened. "Because of the condition of your skin, this may hurt a little, but it will be quick, and then you'll be done."

Within minutes the casts were ready. I gripped the railing on either side as David tugged on the white shells while I tried to keep still. He was right. It was uncomfortable for a few seconds, and then it was over. Perfect replicas of my legs were now in David's hands, and his team at the lab would use them to build me prosthetic legs.

It was my official introduction to an amputee's world; one where I learned what liners, sleeves, pylons, and titanium were, and how that should matter to me. I learned the word prosthetic, which was a bit of a tongue-twister compared to fake, artificial, or peg leg, which conjured images of pirates with eye patches forcing people to walk the plank. I had an official title, which was a bilateral below-knee amputee.

When I was unconscious during the weeks after the crash and infection was raging in my body, my right knee was threatened, and the surgeons were talking about further amputation—a choice they hoped they wouldn't use. I knew having my knees was a huge advantage for an amputee. I needed all the joints I could get.

There was a lot to take in, a lot to accept. When being handed unfamiliar words along with thick squishy liners, I realized the permanence of my situation.

I can't fight this.

I'm changing.

I'm changed.

I held my liners and stared at my inevitable surrender.

Stump was a word I did not like, and refused to use.

Although my prosthetist didn't use the term, many people did. Instead of legs or arms or limbs it was stumps, which brought up words like hacked and dead and rotting...not the images I wanted associated with me. I already had burnt, scarred, MRSA positive, and amputee on the growing list of things that had gone wrong. The last thing I wanted was to refer to my legs as stumps. They deserved more dignity. *I* deserved more dignity. I had legs...legs that still had some ability. They had feeling and bent at the knee. They were a part of me. Stump got stuck in my throat, and never came out. To me, it was a dirty word.

~~~

It was a few weeks before I saw my man-made legs that would join the rest of me and enable me to walk. My legs were inserted into plastic shells called sockets. The sockets were on top of metal pylons, and at the end of the pylons were my new feet. They looked enormous. They *were* enormous.

These legs looked like they weighed as much as I did, and I hoped I wouldn't tip over in them. Their bigness was to accommodate the thick liners I had to wear over my legs. I needed as much cushion as possible to protect my skin. After all, it wasn't exactly ideal to cover my legs with non-porous materials like silicone and acrylic that wouldn't let my skin breathe.

Gail gave me instructions. "You can put your legs on for short periods of time and get a feel for them. You need to stay in bed, though. You're not quite ready to make contact with the floor, yet."

Gail made it a priority to visit me each day and tip the bed slightly so I was slanted, with legs down, not quite vertical. The idea was to allow my body adjustment time to get used to having my legs beneath me, supporting me, rather than straight out in front of me. I had not been upright in five months.

Even though I was only wearing my prosthetic legs for just minutes at a time, we had to be careful to not damage my skin further. We were trying to get that quarter-sized wound on my knee reduced and closed. After "exercising," my prostheses were removed and left to rest against the foot of my bed.

One evening, I was finally given permission to stand and make contact with the floor. Nervous with anticipation, I wanted to get my first steps over with. I wanted to be miles ahead in my recovery, to be on my thousandth step. It was time.

Gail brought in an aluminum walker. My nurse, Ann, came in and together they put on my legs for me and helped me to a sitting position. Gail lowered the railing on the left side of my bed, and I shuffled over to the edge of the bed and moved my legs one at a time over the side, each of them landing with a thunk as they met the floor. The blood rushing to my legs inside the sockets prickled like they were falling asleep. They placed the walker in front of me, each holding an arm, and lifted me to a standing position. My mom was there ready with a camera.

My feet met the floor. *I'm upright.*

I took a breath, and gripped the walker, while Gail and Ann stood protectively on either side of me.

I'm standing.

After long, long months of surgery, and recovery, and enduring, I could feel the floor beneath me. I heard the click of the camera as my mom snapped a photo of my first step, marking my first steps in the same way when I was a baby. I smiled for her.

It was new, but there was sameness to it. It still felt as though I had feet attached to me. My brain recalled my ghost feet. I knew what it was to walk, how to put one foot in front of the other. Like a toddler though, I wasn't strong enough to hold myself up. And I had to learn in cumbersome legs that felt utterly foreign to me. My body recognized the abnormality and wanted to shake them off. But I'd been waiting for this moment, so I ignored the instinct and concentrated on moving my feet forward. It was easier than I thought it would be, and I breathed a sigh of relief that I could do this. I was already further along than I was seconds ago. Finally, finally free from my bed, I felt a surge of strength. I felt more like myself.

I inched the walker out in front of me, and as I did, I took a small step. Then, another step.

The walker supported a lot of my weight, so these tentative steps weren't too strenuous. Since I had no cues from my brain, I looked at my feet as I walked. The floor felt slippery, wavy underneath me, and I relied on my eyes for balance as I walked out of my room and just past the doorway.

I had been in this room for months, and I had just walked to the other side, of my own will, and my own strength. I only took about five steps, but I did it. It was the first time in a long time that I wasn't wheeled or lifted out. It was my first strike for reclaiming independence.

I waited for a rush of emotion, that feeling of being a character in a movie, with the dramatic swell of music, a triumphant fist in the air, and tears streaming down the heroine's cheeks. I should have felt victorious or elated. What I felt was determined because I knew I had a long way to go. I looked at the wide space around me, the hallways I had to conquer, and I saw that the race had only begun and it was going to be a slow, measured one. I couldn't set the pace. Instead, my skin and time would dictate what I could and couldn't do. This wasn't the set of a film, and I wasn't playing a part. I had work to do. This was one first of many firsts. I walked, and I would do it again.

~~~

Each day I took more steps moving past my room's doorway to the nurse's station, and beyond to the waiting room. I was frail, and it took a lot of effort to walk, but I had small goals I wanted to reach within the walls of the hospital. Walker in hands, I walked as much as I could, when I could.

Once afternoon, Scott came to visit, and I wanted to surprise him by walking to him. The nurses were in on my surprise and asked him to wait in the waiting room. As I made my way, I attempted to turn a corner and lost my footing. Before I could recover, before I knew what happened, I landed on the floor. Unable to get up, and unable to help myself, I felt my pride and confidence melt away. Gail swooped in with a wheelchair and, suddenly, the arms and hands of nurses were everywhere, octopus-like, reaching out to scoop me up and ease me into the chair. Tears filled my eyes as I ground my teeth. I felt like a child, dependent and weak. I couldn't pick myself up. I didn't want help. I was so sick of help. I despised how needy I'd become.

Without a word, Gail wheeled me to my room and helped me onto the bed. Her voice was soft and kind. "Do you want to take a few minutes and then walk over to Scott, or would you rather have him come to you?"

"I'll walk. I just need a little time."

"Okay, I'll get the walker." She patted my hand and left. Ensconced within the walls of my room, I was safe, my face flushed with exertion and humiliation. There had been witnesses to my neediness, people to feel sorry for me. *The poor burnt amputee fell.* I was a spectacle.

I pressed my cool hands to my blazing cheeks. "Enough!"

Gail returned with the walker and, once again, chin held high, I began to walk to the waiting room.

Scott was flipping through a magazine and stopped when he saw me. "There you are. Look at you, up and walking!" He came to stand in front of me. "I wondered what happened to you. The nurses told me you were on your way a while ago now."

"I fell."

He grimaced. "Are you okay?"

"Yeah," I exhaled. "I wanted to surprise you, and now I'm just embarrassed." With that admission all the adrenaline left and I was hit hard by fatigue. "Do you want to go back to my room? I'm tired."

Scott met my eyes. "It's still a surprise. I'm proud of you. You should be proud of you." He reached out to touch my arm.

"Don't touch me!" I laughed. "I'll probably fall over."

It felt good to be understood, and relieved I didn't have to delve into a long explanation about being mortified. I should be proud of all that I'd achieved, but all I could think about was what I hadn't done yet and how far I still needed to go. Now, in this moment, as Scott's steps matched my own, his pride could be enough for both of us. It had to be. Together we walked to my room.

~~~

The next day a patient stopped me on the other side of the unit, just outside her room. She looked at me in her wheelchair and said, "You're so lucky."

I didn't know what to say. I blinked. Once. Twice.

She turned to Gail, who was with me, and asked, "Do you think that would work for me?" She was in a wheelchair, her legs bent at the knee and unmoving. She was paralyzed.

Gail gently squeezed her shoulder, "Honey, you don't have the same injuries. Heidi can feel her legs."

It was fascinating to me that our expectations in the hospital and our standards for what we desired were so different from what they may have been on the outside, in the real world, before tragedy found us. What we had in common here was pain. Within the pain, there was a hierarchy. If you had cheated death, that was considered a big deal. The longer your stay at the hospital, the more reverence you were given. If the number of surgeries was high, eyes widened with respect. If you had a spinal cord injury, you would trade places with me in a heartbeat.

The words, *you are so lucky*, found me again. A lovely girl in the room next to me had severe burns to her face and hands, and she said, "You're so lucky it wasn't your face."

I nodded. *Yes, I suppose it is.*

I quickly learned it didn't help to compare. I longed to say, "But you have your feet." Like that was enough explanation for how I didn't feel so lucky, how neither of us was lucky. I couldn't imagine what she had, and what she would always have to endure. She was right in some ways. In the future, I would be able to hide most of my scars, my legs. Her face would always be exposed. We could have gone around in circles with our comparisons, but we would only hurt one another, and we knew we were on the same side.

My very good friend, Loraleigh, told me that no one is an expert on pain. I held fast to that. To say that someone's pain is greater or less than our own was to pass judgment. We were equals in suffering. We should be allowed to feel our pain without someone stepping into it and steering it, telling us how awful or amazing it all was. I knew I needed to be in it, right in the middle of my pain, to see clearly and know what to hold onto, what to throw away and what to hope for.

~~~

My prosthetist thought it would be a good idea for me to meet another bilateral amputee, like myself, but further along in her recovery. She was in a bus accident twenty years ago, and I was allowed to ask her anything I wanted. She didn't normally do this, but she was doing it as a favor to David. She had moved on and didn't like dredging up the past.

When she walked in I paid close attention to her, the way she walked, the way she sat on my bed. She didn't walk like a penguin or with a limp. She moved swiftly, with purpose. She didn't look like an amputee.

I watched her face as she spoke, searching for traces of sadness. When I opened my mouth to ask her questions, I was surprised by what came out. I didn't ask about her accident. I didn't ask about how she coped. I wanted to know, "Can you just lie down on a couch with your legs on? Or do you take them off when you want to relax? Do you go for walks? For how long? How do you shower?" I fired off rounds with my eyes closed and prayed I'd hit my mark. *What would she say?*

I couldn't ask if she still struggled with her accident and the loss of her limbs. I didn't want to imagine myself twenty years later still at the mercy of what happened. I wanted to know if life ever got easier. Did her prosthetic legs become a part of her, or was she still living in a shadow?

I learned that she hiked, kept her legs on when she relaxed on the couch, and used a bath bench to shower. She was busy, active, and I liked the picture she painted. She had truly moved on with her life, and more than that, she *had* a life. She didn't come in hunched over, crippled by her loss. She was thriving, apparently happy, and I resolved I would be that, too.

I imagined myself walking; face lifted to the sun, arms swinging, aware of the rise and fall of my chest as I breathed in and out, listening to the birds calling from the trees. It was summer in my reverie and I was content. I was normal.

11

Hospital Dating

On October 17th, I celebrated my 24th birthday with friends, family, nurses, and a heap of food. My mom was at the helm organizing, directing, and encouraging everyone to eat, eat! It didn't matter that I was flat on my back in a bed. Wherever a group of people was gathered, a feast must be had. We were never short of food growing up in my house. Seconds were always pushed at dinner. If we were full, that was accepted, but not before we were asked if we wanted more. It was no different in the hospital.

My mom stood by my bed, hands on her hips. "Heidi, what would you like to eat?"

I still found eating hard. I had been fed through a tube for so long that food was something I needed to get used to again. "You pick, Mom. You know what I like."

And she was off, launching herself into the next task. My mom was rarely still. All my life she moved—she cleaned, she fed, she looked after. My brothers and I were safe in a love that never stopped.

The crash was especially hard on her. She was at home when it happened; seconds after Betty and I left she heard a bang. *The loudest bang I ever heard* she said, and didn't say much else. I didn't press her for more. She was helpless, powerless to do anything to save her daughter, or make her well. She was forced to wait at the sidewalk while firefighters lifted me from the ravine. Later, she sat by my bed, wringing her lined, hard-working hands.

There wasn't room for anything sad when my mom gathered and assembled everyone to sing Happy Birthday to me. Family and friends, nurses, physiotherapists, and occupational therapists—the many faces of the people I knew and loved – packed themselves into my small room, some spilling into the hallway.

Burning candles weren't allowed what with all the ready oxygen everywhere, but gifts were stuffed on the tray table beside me. It was a far better sight than my water jug, juice, and vomit trays. (my standby was to bring up whatever anesthesia the doctors had pumped in). My room was transformed with bright, crisp wrapping paper and bags with Happy Birthday splashed across them, filled with colorful tissue. I loved having something pretty near me.

While everyone went to refill their drinks, get cake, and second helpings of food, Scott placed a small blue velvet box into the palm of my hand. "For you."

I tugged at the box and the lid sprang open. Inside was a dainty and delicate white gold ring with a small diamond in the center. I looked at him, surprised. "A ring?"

He shrugged. "It looks like you."

He didn't slip the ring onto my finger. He didn't touch it. He sat cross-legged at the foot of my bed and the ring, still in its box, lay between us in the palm of my hand. "It's a promise ring. It's my promise to you, to be with you. It's the promise of us and a future together. And the promise that things will get better."

I felt my face flush with joy. With shaking hands, I took the ring from its box and slipped it onto my ring finger on my right hand. It wasn't an engagement ring. Neither of us was ready for that, yet. On my finger, with me, was a symbol of hope, and a reminder that Scott was here because he wanted to be here. This wasn't just about me, but about both of us and what we had endured together. I felt known. Cherished.

I didn't imagine my 24th birthday would be celebrated in a hospital. I didn't imagine my 24th birthday at all. I had never been one for thinking too far ahead. In school, in job interviews when I was asked where I saw myself in the next five, ten years, I squinted like I was thinking hard, and made something up. I never had any real vision of myself or for myself in the future. I had feelings. There were feelings of hopefulness and possibility, and that was how I lived my life, present and on the wings of potential.

While I was going through rapid changes in the hospital, the world outside didn't exist for me. It couldn't. I had too much occupying me here. My way of being in the present served me well, but it was beginning to wear thin, and I itched for a plan. We were in the middle of month five and each month felt the same. Slowly improving, I was definitely out of the woods, but the road ahead of me was long, and I couldn't see the end.

Scott and I were having a relationship at the hospital, which, as it turned out, was not the best place to get to know one another. We knew commitment on a level that most people who had just begun dating wouldn't have to experience. We didn't, however, know each other's quirks or the things that could drive us crazy. Everything was new when we were thrust into hell, so the usual getting-to-know-you dating rituals would have to come later.

It was our version of cabin fever. We'd been staring at the same walls and surrounded by the same machines for too long. Scott knew every medicine that trickled in through my IV. He knew which drawer to open to retrieve the vomit trays. He saw my bag of pee that hung over the rail of my bed. Our conversations were few, and when they happened, they consisted mainly of hospital talk.

Scott's job as an electrician kept him busy during the day, so he visited often in the evening. I filled him in on my day. "I had a fever."

Scott, looking at the bag of blood hanging beside me, "Oh, I didn't know you were getting a transfusion today. That explains the fever."

"Do you know they're giving me an anti-depressant? I didn't know. I asked Kathleen what all the pills were for, and she said one of them was my 'happy pill'." My central line had been removed, so I could now take my medicine in pill form.

Scott nodded. "Well, that would make sense."

After debriefing, I asked, "What did you do today?"

"Honestly, I don't feel like talking. It's been a long day."

He looked tired, sad. I patted my bed. "Here, come on in. Lie down with me."

All my visitors, including Scott, had to wear gowns and gloves because of MRSA. We needed to be protected from each other. Romance was Scott slipping the gloves off his hands and climbing into the bed to spoon me.

~~~

We had our first fight at the burn unit. It began when he grew frustrated that I couldn't turn myself over in my bed. It was something I had been working on; summoning all the strength I had to move my body from one side to the other. For the first few months in the hospital nurses and orderlies turned me in my bed. He didn't understand why I couldn't just turn to the side and stay on my side. I didn't understand it either, but I was that weak, and Scott couldn't comprehend it.

Months of life and death issues took their toll. My feeble attempts weren't enough for him. "Why can't you roll over?"

"I don't know!"

"Just do it."

He had this calm that irritated me, like if I just applied myself I'd be fine. "Ummm, I've had about a million surgeries, and I'm tired, and I don't know why I can't do it. You do it!" My inability to roll over had a lot to do with missing feet. Feet do a lot of work for you, and when one is used to having them, it takes a while for the body to adjust. I figured that out later.

Scott wasn't a monster. We were tired. The fight wasn't at all about me being able to turn or not turn over. It was all about the fact that we had been there for months, and our relationship was relegated to a room in a building we couldn't escape. It was a lot some days.

When we began to have conversations that bordered on getting to know each other apart from the trappings of the hospital, Scott remarked, "You're a little weird. Have you always been weird, or is that new?"

"Yes!" I almost shouted. It made me smile. I hadn't lost my personality after all, and that included a little weird. I was relieved. So much was influenced by the crash, and it was refreshing to have thoughts and quirks apart from tragedy.

~~~

The months ran into each other, October blurring into November. It was now month six of my stay, and I was given permission to go outside for the first time. The nurses warned me that it might be disorienting, I might feel like turning around. However, I should resist the urge and get outside the walls for a while.

I didn't understand what they meant, not when fresh air swirled around me, not when crisp wind fell on my face. There was staleness in my room that couldn't be helped. Windows didn't crack open on my floor. While I could see the top of the building next to me through the window and know whether the sky was gray or blue on any given day, I never felt what it was like out there.

The days ended early in November, and it was cold. Winter was just around the corner, so I was wrapped in blankets and stuffed into my hospital-issued wheelchair.

Scott leaned against the chain link fence of the deserted tennis courts near the hospital, and faced me. We were silent, neither of us having much to say, content to be alone. It was our first outing in almost six months.

I began to understand the nurse's caution and the urge to return to the walls of the hospital. I had forgotten what outside was, how open and distant everything felt, like the wind would swoop me up at any moment and carry me away. I was a speck in a very big, very wide world. As patients, we were cocooned in the hospital, nestled in a safe, sterile environment. I wasn't sipping margaritas poolside at a resort, but I was in the perfect condition for survival. I was an infant cooed and fussed over, the object of everyone's attention. For better or worse, it had become home.

Even though the hospital was situated in the middle of one of the busiest streets in Vancouver, it was far from the real world. There, on the tennis courts on a frigid night, I saw I was on the edges of that world, the closest I had come to it in a long time. I felt as though I had aged a hundred years, and was afraid of what life out there meant for me. I was ripped from my world as one person, and returning as someone else. *Who would I be now?*

I hooked my fingers in the chain link fence and took in the night. A few seconds passed before I pushed on the tires of my wheelchair. I looked up at Scott, "I want to go home."

12

Home for Christmas

My occupational therapist handed me swatches of fabric in different colors. "Some people get them in bright colors."

Hot pink and electric blue was not going to make this appealing.

I had been here for six months and my skin was healing and toughening up, which meant I was ready for pressure garments. When worn, they apply pressure to scars, flattening and smoothing them out. I chose white and black. Basic, boring, like I was going into battle. I stretched out to be measured, and would receive the garments in a few weeks.

They were like long underwear, but clingy and elasticized. They looked like bad workout wear that was too thin and showed off every bump and flaw. They started at just below my boobs, covered my torso, and stopped at the knee with a zipper along the side, so I could wriggle into them. I was also measured for long sleeves for my arms, made up of the same fabric. I had one small graft on the inside soft part of my arm, not enough to warrant pressure garments. But with all their unmarred skin, my arms had become prime donor sites. Skin was shaved from them often and, eventually, they were as red, purple, and bumpy as the rest of me.

I was consumed with how hot I would be in the summer months straitjacketed like this. Wherever my skin was grafted, I didn't sweat, so I had trouble cooling down once I got hot. A fan set at the highest setting blew air in my room for this reason. My face was often red and flushed, overworked. I was assured that the garments were made of breathable fabric. Uh-huh. I will be wearing clothes on top of clothes, and clunky legs made up of material that doesn't breathe at all.

I felt sorry for myself.

I understood they would be instrumental in healing my skin, going from purple and red to lighter shades of purple and red, then blanching to pink and white. "Do you think it's possible for the garments to take away my scars entirely?" I asked. This might give me more incentive to wear them. Maybe I was crazy, but I continued to hope for miracles.

No, the garments couldn't do that. But they would fade and flatten the scars. I had to wear them for two years every day and night in order for them to do their job, only taking them off to shower.

One quiet evening after I had gone for a short walk around the unit, I lay on my bed, legs still on, when a nurse poked her head into my room. She wiggled a bottle of nail polish at me. "For your toes!"

My depression must have permeated the hallways. Friends and family visited, but I didn't do much to hold up my end of the conversation because I never had anything new to report. I had little to do, but watch TV, which kept me distracted. But nothing dominated my days, so I was numb. I was dutiful and smiled and did what was required of me, but I was on my way toward apathy, and my nurse was about to run interference.

Covering all the metals that made up my feet was a rubber shell made to look like a foot. It was a mannequin foot, perfectly formed, free of flaws and proportioned model toes.

I waved her in. She slapped the bottle against her palm a few times and unscrewed the lid. She took my shoes off, plopped down at the edge of my bed and painted my rubber stuck-together toes the most sparkly silver nail polish I had ever seen.

They were pretty. I was a princess with a new crown. I rarely painted my toenails when I had them. I had long, skinny toes I didn't care to show off. Now, I wished I had loved them more and appreciated them for all that they'd done for me.

My nurse was like a proud mama after that, showing off my painted toes to everyone who came through my door. "You have to see her toes!" *Take pride in your feet, Heidi.* She reminded me of the old Sunday school song, *this little light of mine, I'm gonna let it shine.* And through her, my feet did shine.

~~~

Tinsel, wreaths, and garlands with red berries began to appear on doorways and walls. Themed trees representing the wards of the hospital decorated the lobbies and cafeteria. Little red fire trucks hung from the Burns and Plastics tree. There was a spring to people's steps. Happy complaints of how there was never enough time were heard in the hallways. Christmas was near and people were excited.

December marked month seven of my stay at the burn unit and I discovered I was the first patient to have stayed this long. I hadn't been home yet because I hadn't been stable enough. There was talk of sending me home, back to Abbotsford, for Christmas.

All that changed on Christmas Eve, when I was scheduled to make my first trip home. The morning arrived with snow that had fallen hard in the Lower Mainland. We can have entire winters where we might just get a dusting of snow before the rain washes it away. Snow tends to stay on the mountains, where it belongs, but every other winter, or so, snow covers the mainland and we've never been very equipped for it. We understand rain coming down so hard our windshield wipers can't keep up, but snow dumbfounds us.

Morphine was measured and poured. A bed was ordered for the basement of my parents' home, where I'd be sleeping. Everything was being looked after in preparation for my return home, but the snowstorm had changed everything, which meant someone needed to drive me home. My parents had planned on driving, but the roads were too slick and hazardous. We needed someone with a truck that could handle the snow. The drive from Vancouver to Abbotsford was only about an hour long, but was dangerous.

Calls were made. Who could help? The staff had gone through so much to get me home, and they were going to keep calling until someone said yes. A firefighter named Peter Hansen stepped up and promised to take me home.

My memory of the journey was jerky, snapshots I could barely hang onto. Many hands slid me into the cab of the truck where somebody had the foresight to make me a bed.

Shouts of goodbyes and wishes of a merry Christmas.

The smell of outside, crisp and clear, for a heartbeat.

Blankets pulled up to my chin.

White swollen sky rolled by me as I lay in my makeshift bed. Snowflakes landed on the window, a blanket of stars.

I was going home.

A camera crew was waiting in my driveway when I arrived. I'd been asked earlier that morning, among the flurry of footsteps and hands, if that was all right. In a haze of morphine and activity, I said, "Sure, that's fine."

But, it wasn't fine. I was out of the truck and in my chair when a microphone appeared at my lips. "How do you feel?"

I barely felt the words as they left my mouth. "I'm good, fine. It's Christmas. Happy to finally be at home."

While it was an incredible gift to be home, I wasn't happy. Full of morphine and heartache—life was never going to be the same. I had arrived home with a new body and new eyes. This was the last place I was whole, and the last time I saw Betty. What was I thinking as I got into the car, when Betty closed the door? Were we bright-eyed and chattering about our day? "What did you do today? How are you? Did you get everything packed?" Did we scream when the speeding car came for us? Did we have time to look at each other, one final glance that said we were in this together? Or was it all too fast as my car hurtled toward the chain-link fence?

I shivered. "I'm cold."

Scott pushed me toward the garage. The interview was over.

A few hours later, Angela helped me into a black sleeveless dress she bought for me with money my parents had given her. She brushed make-up on my face and stepped aside as I swung my heavy legs over the side of the bed in preparation to stand. My walker waited for me as I stood, the hem of my dress falling to the floor. I looked up and smiled for my mom as she snapped a photo.

My dad and Scott fashioned a blanket into a sling to carry me up the stairs. It was too awkward to be in someone's arms. My skin was stretched so tight that I felt like I could pop. I was gently lowered into my wheelchair that sat in the living room.

Christmas Eve was something my family had always put more emphasis on than Christmas Day. We'd go to church with our best clothes on, where the lights were dimmed and the tall tree in the corner was aglow with strings of light that wound all the way to the top to greet the angel from her perch. The service was kept short to accommodate families needing to take their young children home and put them to bed, and for families like ours that raced home to open gifts. Christmas Day was a day for lounging and playing with whatever Santa brought the night before.

As I sat in my chair on Christmas Eve, taking in the tree, the carefully wrapped presents placed just so, the faces of my family, and the trays of chocolate and nuts on the coffee table, I wondered if my parents were trying to fill the emptiness that lurked everywhere in the wake of the crash. We were in a room filled to bursting. We talked and talked, punctuating our conversation with laughter, keeping silence at bay, not letting it settle over us. Quiet brought forth our thoughts, and nobody wanted to think. Not tonight.

Friends and neighbors dropped by to visit. Another trip was made with me on top of the blanket, where I was returned to the basement and deposited on my bed. I thought about one of my visitors, a man who attempted to rescue me from my burning car. Shawn had climbed down the ravine to pull me from the wreckage, which proved to be futile, so he stayed with me. He was another piece of the day I was missing, and I was sure I had been told the incredible story of the Good Samaritan who risked his own life to save mine, but I didn't remember. I'd thanked him and, looking back that night, I'd wished I had said more to express my gratitude, but I was dizzy with morphine and the arduous day. The right words had escaped me.

Later, people gathered around my bed in the basement to watch the news. My story was one of the top stories in Vancouver news that night. They talked about the heroic firefighter who braved the snowstorm to bring a burn survivor home. I wished the story had stopped there, but they went on to survey the site of the accident. As the camera swung over the ravine where my car had landed upside down almost seven months ago, tears slid down my face.

"Stop this," I whispered. "I can't do this. Stop it."

The crushed fence, the memorial of crosses and flowers vanished from the screen. My mom's hand was on my shoulder, my shaking body soothed by her touch. One by one, people left until it was just me, my mom, and Scott. At risk were my months of self-preservation, of sticking to survival. There were depths I hadn't reached yet, doors to emotions which had remained shut tight. The evidence of Betty's death was in front of me and grief was a breath away, about to be unlocked, only I wasn't ready to break it open.

My mom smoothed the blankets over me. "It's okay, Heidi. You're tired. Everyone's going. It will be better tomorrow." She kissed me on the cheek and left Scott and me alone.

Lights were switched off and a hush fell over the house as everyone made their way to bed. Scott was going to sleep over on the couch next to me. Tucked in to my automatic bed, the head of it tilted up, Scott climbed in and curled up next to me, his arms around me. I turned to face him and we kissed.

No one was going to check on me. No voices interrupting over crackling intercoms. Outside, snow fell quiet and soft. It was dark as Scott's hands ran over me. I felt whole under his hands, as if I was being put back together. Healing.

The next evening, on Christmas day, I waited to be picked up by ambulance to return to the hospital. With the snowstorm over, the roads had been mostly cleared, making it safe to drive. Just as the ambulance pulled in to our driveway, my friend Lily ran in through the open garage. Breathless with excuses, she came to stand by me at my bed, her cheeks flushed with cold. The paramedics wheeled over a gurney. Her hands fluttered and waved, making up for what she couldn't say.

I felt my dad's impatience as he paced, moving from room to room. She thrust a card and a container filled with fresh-baked cookies at me. Lily made the best cookies.

"Thanks Lily. I'm glad you came by." I didn't know what to say. Lily and I had been friends since we were teenagers. I was friends with her older sister before her, and somehow Lily and I grew to be closer, yet I had barely seen or heard from her while in the hospital.

She left abruptly, saying, "I have to go, Dan's waiting." Dan was her boyfriend, and he was parked on the street, the truck running.

On our return to the hospital, the paramedic asked me about my Christmas.

"It was good. Different." I smiled and shrugged. There was no point in telling the truth, to explain this ended up being harder than I thought it would be. The drive, talking, visiting, the TV news, and Lily running away from me and our friendship were exhausting. Did Lily feel better now that she had dropped off the cookies? I felt like an item she'd checked off her list, her duty done. I wondered if she would feel a little lighter tonight as she fell asleep. Her burden may have lifted, but I felt heavier, weighted with confusion and sorrow. I was bewildered by her actions, yet I couldn't ask her why she couldn't be here and face me. I wasn't able to go after her.

I craved silence, and I was surprised that I looked forward to the hospital. My home didn't feel like home anymore. Life had gone on without me. Now it was the place two blocks from the scene of the crash, where life was divided into Before and After. I didn't know if I could live here anymore.

I thought about firsts, how they were supposed to be exciting, anticipated. I couldn't look at my first surgery, first steps, and now the first Christmas with fondness. These weren't memories I would fawn over later with a glass of wine. These were firsts I wanted to rush through and forget, but it was impossible to put oceans between me and something that hadn't yet faded, and wasn't a memory. The firsts had to happen, and I had to face them. While it was good to be with Scott and my family, I was glad the first Christmas was over.

13

Alone

I approached the end of my seven month stay at Vancouver General. I would be moved out of the burn unit and in to G.F. Strong Rehabilitation Center in Vancouver. It was time to begin the New Year somewhere else.

I grew more and more anxious as the time drew near. While I needed to be on my own and gain physical strength, I was afraid to approach the real world. Rehab meant I was mere steps away from reality, of a long life with disability. I was apprehensive about a new environment and a new reality where my survival skills would be put to the test. I would have to do more than exist. Towards the end of my time at the burn unit, I began to help with my dressing changes, so my army of nurses was no longer needed. Instead, I had one nurse who would wrap my arms. Before she made her way to my room, I unwound the gauze from my arms. It wasn't so much that I was being helpful, but exercising my will, needing to wean myself from constant care.

The staff at VGH had become family, and they knew my needs as well, if not more than I did. I had been in their care for seven months. Meant to foster independence, G.F. Strong was a halfway house to the real world. My nurses and Gail had talked up the center for weeks before my departure. *There's physiotherapy, and a pool, and activities! There will be others like you there!*

It was an opportunity to gain my independence and learn to walk with a physiotherapist who primarily cared for amputees. I wanted to get on with my life, and it was definitely time to go, but I didn't feel ready. I wouldn't be contained in a small room anymore. My boundaries would expand and my drugs would be reduced. I wouldn't have morphine to keep me numb, and I wondered how much I would feel now that the drug wasn't there to flatten me. Would my feelings attack me, razor sharp?

Wheels locked, secure and strapped down, I sat in the back of a van built and designed to transport people in chairs. My legs were in a bag strapped to my chair. My parents were meeting me at rehab, along with the few belongings I had. I wondered if I should get used to getting around this way, in a van for the disabled, as we wound our way through the city. I stared out the window, watching buildings and cars fly past, gripping the arms of my chair, wide-eyed at the prospect of more change.

~~~

At the front desk, I listened to the receptionist at G.F. Strong. "You'll be on the third floor. It's the brain injury floor."

Home would be on the brain injury floor. The brain injury floor. They needed to come up with something cheerier.

Upon registration, I learned testing was required when one is taken to the brain injury floor.

"I don't have a brain injury." My fingers grazed the healing donor site on the right side of my bald head. An infection required my head to be shaved shortly before I left the hospital. "I mean, I know I look like I have a brain injury, but I don't have one. My injuries are everywhere but my head." I waved my hand dismissively and laughed.

She looked at me kindly. My explanation fell on deaf ears. Anyone staying on the third floor had to have their mental capacity tested.

A nurse appeared at the doorway and pushed my wheelchair towards the elevators in the main lobby. The elevators looked like freight elevators, and were wide and large enough to carry a boat-load of people, their chairs, and a small car.

We made our way to the third floor and entered a room filled with round tables, some that held food and objects that reminded me of children's toys. A few people were sitting at each of the tables. Vacant eyes were locked into heads cocked at odd angles. Despair caught in my throat, and I clutched the arms of my chair while looking wildly behind me. I wanted to run.

My chair rolled again, and I was pushed to one of the tables with food. A nurse was careful to pronounce each syllable as she looked at me. "Can you eat the food in front of you?" She put a spoon on the table, as though I would have trouble with it, and asked if I could pick it up.

Fighting back tears, I forced words out of my mouth, "This is a mistake. I'm fine. They've put me here because of the lack of space on other floors. They didn't know where to put me."

She nodded. She glanced at the spoon and said, "Try to eat."

I swallowed hard. "I can eat. With a fork."

"After you take a bite, make sure to swallow your food. We're doing something called a swallow test."

A swallow test? I looked around me again, wanting to scream. "I'm not like them!"

Couldn't she see me? *Invalid* floated through my mind.

She waited as I picked up the spoon, scooped up food and lifted it to my mouth. She watched me closely and scribbled on a sheet of paper.

I didn't know what to do. I had just arrived, and I was already invisible. After a few more questions, yet another nurse came over. She must have seen the exchange because, much to my relief, she said, "I'm sorry. You shouldn't have been brought to this room. Let's get you on your way."

She wheeled me to my room towards the end of the hall. At the door, I forced myself to keep calm. "Thank you. I'll be fine now."

I wanted to cry alone.

The door was ajar, and the tires of my wheelchair squeaked on the shiny floor beneath me as we wheeled inside. The room was simple; a countertop with a mirror above it, a bed, and a large window. I wheeled over to it and checked out the view.

My window overlooked a parking lot filled with vans and buses, people in wheelchairs, on crutches, and wearing halos (a brace that prevents your head and neck from moving). Some were smoking, some were being loaded onto a bus, and some were just arriving, like me. They were in unknown territory. We all were. We were here linked by tragedy, bad luck, and our differences. I sat in my wheelchair and I felt it—the enormity of my differences settling in the pit of my stomach. I had never felt more alone.

Invalid followed me into the room.

A knock on the open door startled me. My parents. My mom patted my shoulder and pressed her cheek to mine, murmuring, "Don't cry." My dad handed me a teddy bear, a satin heart stitched to its paws. We looked like the people in the parking lot. I was shell-shocked and lost. "I just want my legs back."

I needed for them to go. And Scott would be here within minutes. I needed to be alone for a while, so I smiled through my tears. "I'll be okay. It's a long drive back home, and there'll be traffic." *Just go, go. I'll see you soon.*

When they left, I stayed at the window and stared at my future. I whispered to the window, "God, if you can hear me, if you see me, please make my life count for something. I'm here. Please. See me."

14

Starting Over

I am walking, running, climbing stairs. I'm like the wind, flying and sailing over lush fields and bodies of sparkling blue-green water, where there is no color, no name for ocean when it looks like this. I can't go fast enough. I am agile and nimble as I take stairs in twos. I feel the weight of my body, the stretch and pull of my calves. I dare myself to leap over three stairs this time. I can do it, and I'm pleased.

There's a sudden pull, a crack in the blue sky above me. I trip. I collide with this world and the next, the one I'm a part of now, forever. I know I'm not in the right body. I turn and all at once everything is awash in gray. Unanchored by feet, my legs are scraping the ground as I run. I'm in an unending field. It's too fast, I'm too fast. The lights are off and I don't know where I'm going.

My eyes snapped open. It's only a dream. I took inventory.

Pat, pat at my legs. My fingers traveled to the large divot in my left thigh and rested there. My legs were too light; where ankles and feet should be, I feel air. I'm unmoored with nothing to keep me tethered to the ground, to the earth. It feels wrong. *I* feel wrong.

The realization of what happened crept along until grief was a blanket suffocating me and pinning me to the bed. After all this time, I was still surprised at the ferocity of grief, and couldn't believe the stranglehold it still held on me. It had been eight months since the crash, and I discovered that grief had layers I didn't know existed. Plagued by nightmares of my legs whole and then shattered, skin perfect and then ravaged, I wondered when they would finally stop. When would I reach the bottom?

The door creaked open. I screwed my eyes shut. I heard the squeak, squeak of shoes meeting clean floor, approaching my bed.

Gray morning light peeked through closed blinds and the nurse spoke softly, "It's time to get up and take a shower."

I opened my eyes and saw there were two nurses armed with a wheelchair designed for the shower. It looked plastic and hard. No sleeping in for me. It was all business.

The nurses easily scooped me up and settled me into the chair. I looked over my shoulder at my prosthetic legs propped up, right and left, side by side, against the bed. They were left behind as I was wheeled briskly out of my room, down the long hallway, past the nurse's station, and into a shower stall. The smell was the same everywhere I went, food and sick covered up with sterile soap. I was helped out of my nightgown while the faucet turned on with swiftly rising steam.

I shivered, cold with the early morning and the awareness that I was showering in a chair while a stranger helped wash me. As water poured over me, emptiness did, too. I felt like a child. Only children or the very elderly or…I stopped. *The disabled*. The disabled need this kind of help. My shoulders slumped. I wanted to bang my fists on the arms of my chair and wail. Who was this girl trapped in a weak, decrepit body?

I was wheeled back to my room, wrapped in sterile white towels that made me itch. The nurses helped me dress, handing me a shirt and threading my prosthetic legs through shorts. Once I rolled my liners over my limbs, they helped put on my legs, and I settled back into my wheelchair. It was a huge ordeal, and I was beat.

"Are you all set then? Do you need anything else, Heidi?"

I nodded, eager for them to go. "No, thank you."

"Breakfast will be here soon and then it's time for physiotherapy. You know where physio is now, right? Do you need help getting there?"

I had been given the tour the day I arrived. I smiled. "I'm good. I know where to go."

I was grateful for their help, but I wished I didn't need help. I ached for independence.

I ate breakfast slowly, taking time to stop and stare at my prosthetic legs. I was still stunned by them and wondered when they would feel like a part of me, *if* they would ever feel like a part of me. Because my skin was still healing, it was sore and sensitive, and it was hard to tolerate stuff digging into it. It didn't take long before wounds were reopened and new wounds were created. But today my fake feet rested on my chair's footrests, and I was determined to begin physiotherapy.

Metal parts attached to bodies walked by me. A young man was stretched out on a floor mat, his prosthetic leg off and resting beside him. A woman unraveled the gauze from her leg inspecting a bleeding wound. These people are like me.

"You must be Heidi." It was my new physiotherapist, Linda. "Heidi, can you walk at all? Can you walk between these bars?"

I nodded my head, eager to please. "I can walk a little."

"Show me."

I wheeled myself to the parallel bars in the middle of the physiotherapy room and pulled myself up. I steadied myself, tugging at my shorts. I walked slowly, sliding my hands along the bars as I placed one foot in front of the other. I kept my eyes on my feet until I reached the end.

"Okay! Good, good. We've got a lot of work ahead of us," she said while wheeling the chair over to me.

I eased myself into my chair and craned my neck toward Linda. "Do you think one day I'll be able to walk well? It's important to me to walk well." I didn't want to look disabled.

She nodded. "That's what I'm here for. Come back tomorrow, and we'll get started."

At noon, with a food tray on my lap, I wheeled over to the table where people and their wheelchairs were parked. I shyly placed my tray on the table and began to pick at the food. I didn't have much of an appetite. Moving on to rehab after seven months in the hospital hadn't done much to cure my lack of appetite. I missed loving food.

It was disconcerting eating with so many people who had fallen upon tragedy. It was astounding to me that each person had gone through life-changing events which brought them to this place, and now we were eating hot dogs together. Forced together because of our injuries, bound by what we had in common.

I don't want to be here. I don't belong here. Immediately struck by guilt, I knew I shouldn't feel this way. I didn't want to be viewed as disabled or different, as they were. Even though my injuries warranted joining a group now, I didn't want to be a part of a group that was judged, or pitied, or ignored.

I *did* belong here, and I hated it.

We were spread out in age, and while picking at my food, I learned this group was the 'second floor clients' (we were called clients, not patients) with spinal cord injuries. Interestingly enough, they were like the popular kids in high school. Most of them were outspoken and tough despite their injuries and insecurities. They doled out acceptance as they saw fit, so I was surprised when they accepted me quickly. Everyone was hurt, wounded by freak accidents or risks they'd taken, and it wasn't surprising that most of the spinal cord clients were young men with wives and families.

"What's your story?"

I looked up. I wasn't sure who asked, but I noticed a few pairs of eyes were trained on me. It was a common question here. Head ducked down, I answered, reluctant to tell it, tired before I began.

It came out in a whoosh, wanting to get it over with. "I was in a car crash. I stopped at the stop sign and went straight through the intersection when another car t-boned us on the passenger side. His car sent my car into a fence, and we landed upside down at the bottom of a ravine."

"Oh my God!"

"That's terrible."

"Where did it happen?"

"It happened right around the corner from my house."

They nodded in unison, knowing. "They say it happens like that. Close to home."

"Was someone with you? Was anyone else hurt?"

"The driver and passenger of the other car walked away just a little banged up. But...my friend..." I swallowed hard. "She died on impact."

Any vitality I had left as soon as this question was asked. I left out details. A few liked to fill in their story with color and anecdotes, leaning forward. Most of us were like me, not so willing, and we rushed through our stories before coming to an abrupt end.

Being rehabilitated became all about what we couldn't do anymore. Or what we wanted to do, but hadn't done yet and now would never be able to do. If I could just turn the clock back by seconds, I could climb that mountain. I could take dance lessons I had never taken, but wished I had.

Suddenly everyone was a skier, a cyclist, and a rock climber. It hurt to see anyone using their legs in a way we couldn't. We had run out of time, and we weren't given notice. No countdown to life as you know it will be over. I was jealous, coveting what I once had.

I met one person at our table who claimed he had few regrets. He felt he'd done plenty. His accident was a result of his own carelessness, and he accepted that. Quadriplegic now, he would always be confined to a wheelchair with hand controls to move him.

"It sucks, but it is what it is," he said, philosophically. "It could have been worse." He flicked the lever on the arm of his chair and sped off.

I didn't know if it could get much worse.

Most of us in rehab were in different stages of grief. Some were still in denial, believing their paralyzed bodies would walk again. Some were angry, wisecracking and fuck you-ing their injuries and everything around them. I was somewhere in between.

Before the car crash I was 5'6" and thin with muscular legs and strong arms. I had a toned, flat tummy, which now puckered and bunched due to grafts, and a long red scar that ran right down the middle. I had a twenty-three-year-old body, in good shape, skin hard and soft in all the right places. I ran. I walked. I hiked. I rarely stopped moving. And I had suddenly aged, my skin sagged and drooped where it hadn't hardened with surgery. I joked that my butt had burnt off. Completely grafted, the skin was so thin, it was difficult to sit for any real length of time. I could handle maybe an hour of sitting, even with a specially designed cushion, but I often excused myself to go lie down and take the pressure off my bony bum.

My body was a collection of thick, raised scars, slashes of purple and red, thin rice-paper skin that broke easily, open wounds stubbornly refusing to heal. Repulsed by my body, I made sure to avert my eyes when I passed a mirror. I didn't know what to do with the changed girl trapped in a reflection.

A guy who looked to be around my age was talking now. "Well, I'm outta here by the end of the week."

I was bold, bolstered by our story-telling, "Are you worried about going home?" I wanted to ask if he was scared, like me. But I thought it was too much, maybe too intimate of a question to ask of someone I just met.

"No, I've been here long enough. It's time to go." He seemed confident, resolute. He didn't *need* to be here anymore. "It's easy to get stuck. It's important to do whatever it takes to go home." He looked right at me.

My eyes slid to the plate in front of me, concentrating on the half-eaten hot dog and a small puddle of ketchup. He grabbed his tray, set it on his lap and wheeled deftly to the long counter.

The cafeteria quieted. Lunch was over and almost everyone at the table left. I deposited my unfinished food at the counter and wheeled to the elevator to return to my room. Visitors were coming.

15

Disabled

"You're still you," Scott said while sitting on my bed across from me, focused on my well-being. Heels dug in, determined I'd see that I was still here. I nodded at him, not wanting a fight.

Yes, I was still me *and* I'd lost a body that carried and housed me for twenty-three years.

Offered as comfort, people often confided they had parts of their body they didn't like. I never knew what to do with that. So they didn't like their chubby arms or the long scar on their knee. So what? Their bodies weren't ravaged by fire, their lives turned inside out. I walked a fine line between acceptance and denial, and I worried about being forever lodged in the middle, in grief.

"I don't know who I am, Scott. I just want to be better. I want to stop feeling like this."

"Like what?"

I brought my hands to my chest. "Sad. Numb. Lost. I don't know. Everything." I shook my head, "Let's go outside."

"Do you want to really get out of here?" he asked. "We could go for a drive."

I hadn't been in a car, yet. I had been in a bus, in the truck to go home for Christmas. I hadn't just gone for a drive, devil-may-care. The idea had merit. "Okay. I have to sign out."

In Scott's car, we wound through downtown traffic. "Does it scare you? Being in a car?"

"No. Surprisingly, I'm good. I thought I'd be scared, but I'm okay. I think it's because I don't remember anything about that day, or the crash. It feels good being out like this."

"Do you want to stop anywhere and sit for a while?" We were close to the beach. People were everywhere walking, cycling, running. Moving.

"Let's keep driving." It was a clear day, a day for going somewhere. I wanted to do that, to run away, to leave this sadness, my body, behind and go somewhere. Anywhere. Sensing I didn't want to talk, Scott turned up the volume of the music. I looked out of the window at the changing scenery and lost myself in 'before.'

I was a late bloomer and spent many years mired in insecurity. In high school, I'd avoided most parties, and wasn't one of the popular kids. I had good friends, but I was confident that life began after high school, and all I had to do is just bide my time.

I was somewhere in between, and for a long time this is how it was with me—in between—neither here nor there. Grades eight and nine were mostly spent along the lockers, in the shadows. I had braces, glasses too big for my face, and a bad perm. In grade ten, the braces came off, and I saw what big teeth I had. Glasses were replaced with contacts, and I lost the perm. It wasn't exactly a makeover out of the movies, where I walked down the stairs in slow motion à la 1987's *She's Out of Control* with Tony Danza, but I got it together a little.

After high school, the most hardcore I got was faking my way into a bar at eighteen and ending up in a light make-out session with some guy I'd danced with for all of five minutes. I got really drunk only once in my early twenties. I just didn't do many spontaneous things that bordered on careless, or what many considered fun. I was good to the bone, made decisions that were right, and if it was a gray area, my decisions at least leaned to the right. I got good grades in school and kept my feelings to myself.

I was very controlled until I wasn't. Somewhere between the ages of eighteen and nineteen I developed an eating disorder. It started out slowly and took on a life of its own. I battled with it for five years. I went to counseling, confided in friends, and did everything I could to rid myself of it. It didn't want to go. It hung on, standing at my shoulder whispering in my ear, a growing giant.

If I listened to the disorder, I was ugly. Since I was nine years old, I'd heard those words in my head. I never knew where they came from. My parents insisted I was beautiful, but I knew better. I was plain, and nothing special. Forgettable. Ugly resided at the back of my mind, clawing its way forward until I gave it my full attention. I used to hit my head with my brush because I deserved it. I pinched and scratched my arms because I could never be enough. I was empty, powerless, and the disorder filled me.

Pain manifested as bulimia, and made for an odd companion. I got so close to it, it was all I knew. It's how I coped. Binge, purge. How would I let it go? What would life be like without it? I didn't know, so I didn't test it. I fed it. Bulimia ruled me, and I was inside-out for it. Pain so buried, I was paralyzed.

I lay on my bed shaking, appalled, defeated. *I can't stop throwing up.*

I understood the dangers of eating disorders. I witnessed it in high school. I had friends who accepted it as part of them, a way of life. I knew better. *I don't want this. I don't know how to stop it. Why, why can't I just end this?* I needed something to do.

I sprung up from the bed and walked the short distance to the kitchen I shared with Angela, my roommate, and began to sweep. It didn't take me long to finish and I moved on to the next task, the bathroom. I scrubbed and wiped until there was nothing left to clean. I surveyed my work, pleased with what I'd accomplished. Just as I was about to search for another distraction, I caught my reflection in the mirror.

I moved closer. I was careful around mirrors. They were meant for scrutiny and inspecting my flaws. I met my eyes. Flat, lifeless. Where did I go?

"Do you want to live?" From deep within, a small voice I recognized as truth.

I knew then that this thing was killing me, if not my body, then my spirit. Out loud I said, "Yes."

I want to live.

Something sleeping stirred and stretched inside me. Something was different today. The air around me shifted. I looked into my eyes again.

I matter.

The small voice spoke again, as if the heavens parted, "You are beautiful."

I had hunted healing for years, and I couldn't find it. Shrouded in shame and secrecy, bulimia had too much power. Maybe today was the day I didn't have to be ugly. Today I could take control.

Week after week, beauty was something I discovered in a quiet place inside myself, and I reached out to it again and again. Beauty could belong to me.

When I felt powerless, I didn't panic. I was solid. I hung onto myself, to that small voice. The giant at my shoulder weakened, unhooking its claws, its weight lifting from me. I returned to my former body, the one that knew when it was full and knew when it was hungry. I didn't have to be afraid of emptiness. I acknowledged it and accepted it. I learned to cope. Confronted with feelings I used to dismiss and pretend didn't exist until I stuck my finger down my throat, I stopped vomiting and began to deal with conflict. I faced my emotions and let them be, giving them space inside me until they were real and I could live from a place of freedom. I didn't see myself through a disorder, through a dark veil anymore. I could see me. There was light behind my eyes and I saw the world anew, like it had been washed clean. I mattered.

That day was made for a miracle, the day I claimed my life.

I had been full of hope.

~~~

Through my window the sky grew dark, the sun dipping behind the mountains. Scott said, "We should probably go back."

I sighed. I didn't take my eyes off the sky. "We should."

I wasn't the person who needed a wake-up call in life. I'd had my wake-up call. I was no longer reckless with my life. My life had been reevaluated, turned over, and I was on good terms with it. I had changed. I toyed with the idea of going back to school. I had begun dating someone I thought I could marry. I worked through some difficult issues, learned how to feel, and faced my life. I was on the brink. Of what, I didn't know, but I felt I was on the brink of something good. Unknown and good.

My body and soul were entwined, impossible to sever. Scott's words came back to me. *You're still you.*

I turned to Scott, picking up the conversation we'd started in my room. "I'm still me, but I'm at the age where I'm supposed to figure out who I am. I'm supposed to 'find myself'." I hooked my fingers in the air making air quotes. "I don't know if I believe in 'finding myself'. I used to find it funny when people said that. I thought it was a cop-out or just an excuse to do whatever the hell you wanted."

I waved my hands around. "Now I feel like I'm cheated out of backpacking through Europe, or deciding on a major, or partying hard, or doing any other clichéd thing that's supposed to give me insight into who I am."

I looked at the sky, inky now with brushstrokes of black and blue. I was 'finding myself' in the aftermath of a car crash.

I returned to my new home, my mind full. As Scott made the hour-long drive home, I lay in bed, desperate to succumb to sleep, desperate to escape my thoughts.

My wounds seeped into my subconscious, my dreams working out what I couldn't, sorting out the confusion and loneliness that went along with this place. Even though I faced my new world each day, I must have ached for a miracle, for a restored life, and in my dreams I wandered among broken bodies and had visions of limbs snapping together, spines straightening, and crippled hands functioning. Under the cover of night I was a healer, filled with hope, only to wake up and come to earth with a dull thud.

Reality didn't come with a bang at rehab. It came slow and steady until I was swallowed by it. Being here was inspiring because I was surrounded by people who wanted to overcome the horrible events that led them to this place. It was heartbreaking because we had to learn to accept every change that came with these horrible events. We were different people now.

At the rehabilitation center and in the city of Vancouver, there were opportunities and activities that were modified to people like me. You could go skiing, rappelling, canoeing! The list was long, and everything could be changed to make it doable for you, the disabled person.

I avoided most group outings or activities, preferring to keep to myself. I was friendly, especially with the second floor clients and the few people I met in out-patient physiotherapy, but I was mostly a loner at rehab.

I had been here for two months, nine months since the crash. I kept my head down and moved through my schedule, the next day the same as the last, when one day I decided it was time to release myself from my self-imposed exile and do something, anything! I signed up to go sailing with a group of people from my floor. I had been sailing before and thought it might be nice to be plunked into the ocean.

One by one we were loaded onto the bus. I could wear my legs today, but I still needed my chair. The latest hits blared through the speakers, and I was grateful for it, drowning out any need for conversation. While I was finally participating, I didn't want to make small talk with anyone, or delve into what happened one more time. *How long have you been here? Where are you from? How long do you have to stay? What happened to you?* I kept my eyes on the window, anticipating the ocean.

I arrived at Jericho Beach, the same beach Scott and I visited days before the crash, where we held hands, where he took my picture, where he washed my feet. I waited at the dock until we were ready to set sail.

I slipped on a lifejacket and gripped the arms of my chair to ease out of my seat to stand. I took the large, soft cushion that came with me everywhere and placed it on one of the boat's seats. *How am I getting in this boat?* Still learning how to maneuver myself and my legs, anything new presented a problem.

Thankful our supervisors were busy helping my fellow trippers, I grabbed the railing and lowered myself to sit on the specially raised seating in the boat. I wanted to try this on my own. All my life I could just sit down, and now my brain worked hard, rerouting how I could sit. I swung my heavy legs over until they landed and, using my hands, I moved them until they were positioned well in front of me.

Yesss!

I stretched out my right leg to relieve my knee, which was still in the process of healing. Because of the prolonged healing time, I was unable to wear my right prosthetic leg as often. But it served me well and, as I ran my fingers along the rim of the boat, I once again reminded myself that I was in a special-needs boat.

My lifejacket acted as a buffer from the wind and saltwater that sprayed in my face as we bumped up and down through the water. No one spoke. The only sounds were the waves crashing against the boat and seagulls' greedy calls from a gray, gray winter sky.

Sitting with my back stiff against the sides, I looked sidelong at the few people with me. I'd avoided them on the bus, and now I couldn't. Aside from the able-bodied person manning the boat, all I could see was misfortune and misery. This man must have had a strong neck once and now his head drooped to one side, the features of a young girl's face were twisted, and a woman's hands lay gnarled and unmoving in her lap. It hurt to look at them. Were they as sad as I was? *I'm one of them now. Disabled. Will I ever get used to it?* I fixed my eyes on the cool blue of the ocean, straining to feel nothing, nothing.

When we returned to shore and headed back to the bus, the gray settled over me, and a chill ran along my spine. I looked out at the horizon where ocean met sky, and what I used to see as limitless and promising, was foreboding. The distance was too great, the ocean, too wide. *Where can I go from here? Who will I be?* I couldn't answer a single question about my future. I didn't dare to ask any. I wanted to scream, but my voice would be swallowed by the wind. The question of "What now?" scratched at my mind, relentless in its bleakness. I was heartbroken.

16
The Un-Fairy Tale

"Bless you."

I rolled my eyes as the elevator doors slid shut.

I sighed heavily, my hands tense on the arms of my wheelchair. I was annoyed at the man in the suit who couldn't help himself, who had waited fifteen flights up to bless me as he exited the elevator. I'm sure he meant well, but I didn't need anyone's blessing.

Now that I was at G.F. Strong, I got out more, maybe not quite in the way I wanted—being hemmed in by appointments at the wound care clinics or leg fittings at my prosthetist—but I had little tastes of freedom by being bused all over the city and making my own way, and left to my own devices.

I left the confines of everything structured to take care of me with increased regularity, which meant I encountered more people, people who didn't know what had happened, and people with sympathy.

I knew what I looked like. In their shoes, *I'd* take a second look. I was a clown in a garish costume in a sea of ordinary, and all I longed to do was to step out of my costume and join the sea. That longing grew greater as strangers went out of their way to place a hand on my shoulder, mutter a quick prayer, or crouch to look me in the eye and ply me with questions.

"What happened to you?"

This was asked with each word enunciated, emphasis on the *you*.

My standard answer was, "I was in a car accident." Instantly, I'd remember it's crash...crash. I'm supposed to say crash, since this was no accident.

For some who understood tight-lipped responses, the answer was satisfactory, and they moved on. Others were immune to social cues, and followed up the first question with wide eyes. "Was it bad?"

I wanted to respond with snark. "Are you kidding me?" followed by, "Seriously??" before finally settling on a look so filled with disdain that I would put a moody teenager to shame. But I opted for the polite way, the painfully polite way, and met their irritating curiosity with calm. "Yes. It was bad."

Disappointment flashed in their eyes before they turned and left. I enjoyed not giving them what they wanted.

Scott and I came up with alternative stories to explain how I lost my legs to the strangers who continued asking. Shark attack, legs slammed in a door, sword fight! Scott was my constant comic relief and a master of the straight face. Sarcasm and a dark sense of humor lent itself well to my situation. The fact remained that my story trumped sword fight or any other story we concocted for our amusement. My story was the kind that kept going. Just when you thought I had reached the worst part, it got worse. Sometimes I just wanted a different story.

There were times, especially when I was in for long appointments, that I didn't mind answering questions. It was easier to take from trained medical personnel. I didn't feel like a freak sideshow. They'd witnessed and cared for plenty of freaks. After we got 'what happened' out of the way, talk of Scott came up, the boyfriend who didn't leave. This was what grabbed people; that he was still here.

One morning I returned to VGH so the occupational therapist could check my pressure garments and see how my skin fared underneath.

"So, you'd only been together six weeks?"

"Yup." She mouthed wow.

I knew what was next because I heard it a lot.

"It's amazing he stuck with you. What a great guy!"

I chewed on my bottom lip and nodded. "He's a good guy."

She shook her head. "Amazing! Does he have a brother?"

He didn't. My responses were always the same, delivered in a bright and chipper manner, "Nope! He's got an older sister."

I laughed because it was expected. While she was struck by my good fortune, I was irked by the picture her words created. I should be grateful for his sticking around because who would ever want me in my state? It was a painful implication.

I didn't want to be with anyone who felt guilted into being with me. It's true—I would have been a tough sell to any guy in his right mind, but I was bothered that Scott was a hero in this scenario, like it had nothing to do with me. He swooped in, a knight on his horse, and rescued me, as if I didn't live this every day.

I didn't care for fairy tales very much, even as a little girl, and always believed that girls were strong enough to get themselves out of their bad situations. Come on, Cinderella, stop scrubbing the floors and leave your evil stepmother and stepsisters. Drop your broom and walk out that door with your head held high! Snow White, you're really going to take a bite out of that apple from a crazy, ugly old witch! Really? Use your head.

Still laughing, I said, "Actually, I'm a catch. He's lucky to have me."

"Oh, I didn't mean that you weren't…"

"I know you didn't. It's just that it gets said a lot, and he *is* a great guy, *and* I'm a good person," I offered as explanation. I beamed with conviction.

Scott and I were honest with each other and not easily offended. If I asked Scott for his opinion, I got it uncensored. When I asked him about all the scars, my hands sweeping through the air over myself to emphasize all the scars, he said, "We're both missing out here. I'd like your body back, too."

I sighed. I didn't like how I looked, so how could he? His acceptance seemed easy, too easy. "Will this matter to you? Maybe not right now, but later. A month, a year from now? I will never have my body back. Are you attracted to me? You might change your mind."

I didn't want to be anyone's burden. We were equals.

His answer was slow and measured, "Sure, the scars are there, but so are you. I love you." He added, with a reassuring smile, "You're still cute, you know. We're going to be okay."

Thinking before speaking, Scott didn't say things he didn't mean. He wasn't here out of obligation. He was here because he wanted to be.

I felt relieved at having said the words out loud. I had to believe I was a catch. If I didn't, who would? Scott was a hero, not because he was my knight in shining armor saving me from disaster, but because he stepped into the disaster with me. He looked past what was ruined and saw me.

17
Still Me

I was eager to move from patient to person. Each day was laid out for me. Physiotherapy, occupational therapy, meals and rest were scheduled. Structuring my days brought some evenness to my life. However, I missed having a life of my own. I was tired of being accountable to a team of people.

Decisions had been made for my benefit since my arrival at the hospital. For ten months my life had not been my own. These decisions saved my life, so I wasn't arguing, but being a patient was like being a child. Lying on your back every day with rails on either side of you, dependent...your brain gets soft.

At G.F. Strong, there was more opportunity to be self-sufficient, to work my way toward independence, but I still moved from one set of arms to another, and decisions continued to be made for me.

In a meeting with my prosthetist, an occupational therapist, a social worker, and my mom, we were discussing my reintegration into the real world and the necessary steps to get me out there and on my own.

I'm sure no one intended to exclude me, but somewhere along the way I was forgotten. She needs, she wants, she should. They were talking about my ability to get around in the future, and I was adrift in the conversation.

"Perhaps it's best for her to have a scooter."

"Heidi isn't able to walk as much as we'd hoped, so..."

"She'll need a large enough van to accommodate a wheelchair or a scooter."

"We'll have to sign her up for driving lessons. She'll need to learn how to use hand controls to operate a vehicle."

I heard myself agreeing just to bring the meeting to an end. "Okay, I'll take the lessons." It wasn't what I wanted, but it would get me driving.

Everyone looked pleased as they shuffled their papers and made their way to the door, but I became agitated. *When did I become a paraplegic?* Hand controls made sense for people who couldn't feel their legs. *When did I turn eighty and need a scooter?* They may as well have put an orange vest on me, attached bells, and slapped a sign on my chest that said, 'I'm Handicapped.'

My brain was soft. I needed to get control, to think for myself. I wasn't where I want to be. Not far enough. Just more of the same. I wanted to snap my fingers and arrive. Ta da! Here I am!

I finished lunch and returned to my room, where I flicked on the radio and rolled to the mirror to do something with my uneven hair. It had grown in thick and almost black, and I was grateful it was coming in at all. I sat tall, shoulders back, and studied myself. As I stared at my reflection, I was overcome with a feeling akin to homesickness. I wanted to go back, to reverse time. I felt stuck.

Music was powerful in those days, where I moved forward so slowly that I wondered if I'd made any progress at all. Any song with meaningful lyrics and a melody that swept me up in its beauty hurt. Top forty was all I could handle, and in 1999, thankfully, there wasn't much that was powerful or moving.

But this day was different. I was swallowed up by music, ambushed on a Monday with Peter Gabriel's "In Your Eyes." It made me want to forget, and I let each note turn into an aching so deep, I didn't know if I could bounce back.

Bounce back.

I liked the way it sounded, but I wasn't so sure I was capable of bouncing back from anything. I had been here for three months. My restoration was sloth-like, inching its way towards freedom, even though I didn't know what freedom would look like if I got there. Would I recognize it when I saw it? Would I wake up one morning, home-free, or would it sneak up, unshackling me a little at a time until I was lighter, happier, and the gap between me and the crash had grown wide enough that I could leave it behind? I suspected it would be the latter.

That day I curled into myself and wept. I needed to remember where I came from...who I am. Spent and disoriented, I looked at the clock above the doorway. It was almost time for my next appointment. Time never stopped, not even for a breakdown.

As a fresh amputee, I came across people who felt it important that I know others with injuries like mine, thinking we would have that in common and be friends. I didn't understand that. Just because we were amputees didn't mean we were immediately bound together, having long meaningful conversations over glasses of wine, forever friends. Sharing similar injuries doesn't necessarily create chemistry.

But there were two women in physiotherapy I especially liked and admired. One was a police officer, Laurie, who had been shot in the leg in the line of duty. This resulted in an amputation below the knee. The other was Gail, who had lost her leg above the knee to cancer. We were in physiotherapy from Monday to Friday, so this was a ripe climate of opportunity to be with other people who understood. We became quite friendly and visited the resident social worker together every now and then. It was a time to talk, to be there for each other and, sometimes, air grievances.

"Do you know what makes me crazy?"

"What?"

"When people say everything happens for a reason."

"Totally."

"Why do people say God won't give you more than you can handle? This is way more than I can handle."

"The other one I can't take is when people say this will make you stronger," Gail said, "or, this will grow your character. What does that mean?"

We were in agreement. What *did* that mean? I'd heard that "growing character" bit more than once. At this point, I figured I had all the character I could handle.

"Do people often tell you how strong you are?" I asked. "I hear it a lot. *You're so strong.* But the truth is I don't feel very strong. The only path I see is the one in front of me. And that path is to keep going. To fight. What else would I be doing? If I want to get better, I have to get up every day, and I have to do what's in front of me, or my life is over. It's tragic enough that this happened, but wouldn't it be just as tragic if I gave up?"

Overcome with weariness, I switched gears. "Okay, one more thing, and then I'll stop talking. I really hate it when people keep asking me if I've tried aloe." With all the medical intervention and the best surgeons in British Columbia working on me, the suggestion that no one had thought to use aloe made me crazy, like it was some super cure. Good for small cuts and superficial burns, not for burns so deep, multiple surgeries were required to save your life. A friend, in my defense, once said, "There isn't a plant or bottle of lotion in the world big enough."

Laurie shook her head and agreed. "People say the dumbest things."

People meant well. The three of us acknowledged that. At a loss for words, we rely on clichés and old advice that was never wise advice to begin with. Coming up with the right thing to say was hard. We wondered why people couldn't stick with "I'm sorry," or tell the truth, "This is terrible." It was always a relief to me when people called it like it was. Even saying, "I don't know what to say" was bearable. Silence offended, too. We didn't need space. We needed our loved ones near us.

We found things in common with each other that went beyond our missing limbs. Our willingness to get on with life, to not give up, and the dumb things people said was what brought us together. From Monday to Friday I could look around the room and take comfort that someone knew what it was like to be me.

18
Sweet Victory

I didn't want an audience. It was noon and almost everyone was in the cafeteria. The few patients outside were near the entrance, smoking or waiting to get picked up for appointments within the city. I stood at the sidewalk, across from a small park, shoulders squared, hands wrapped around the walker in front of me, about to cross the street all by myself.

I had many setbacks during my time at rehab. The quarter-sized wound on my knee had shrunk to the size of a dime, but the skin still refused to knit together. It needed oxygen, so I could rarely wear my prosthetic legs, and no amount of wishing and hoping would get me on my feet.

If it were up to me I would be an unstoppable machine excelling at walking, a force of nature as I defied the odds and sped around on my prosthetics, taking to them like I was born to do this! But my body didn't catch up to my fantasy. It was slow and needed time.

There was progress in other areas. I could sleep on my stomach again. For months I could only sleep on my back or, with help, on my side. Now, I had the freedom and strength to roll over on to my stomach and fall asleep the same way I had since I was a baby. My legs, however, were another matter.

I often watched from the sidelines, envious of other amputees as they got up and moved around the physiotherapy room. They made it look easy, even though I knew that wasn't truly the case. I had to make do with stretching exercises and feeble leg bends, nowhere near the goals I longed to achieve.

Phantom pain was discussed, and I'd wondered about it. *Did I have it? How often? And would I need medication for it?*

I'd originally heard about this strange phenomenon of phantom pain in the hospital and how it struck at any time, coming from a body part that's no longer there. Doctors once believed that it was a psychological problem, but phantom pain actually originates from the brain and spinal cord. When I was at VGH, I never felt a sudden spasm of pain from feet that didn't exist. I was in pain most of the time, and I couldn't separate one kind of pain from another. It was that, or the extraordinary amount of morphine I was given was doing its job.

When I arrived at G.F. Strong, morphine was replaced with Tylenol 3's. I didn't take them. I decided I was done with all pain medication, so I stopped in one fell swoop.

I'd grown weary of medicine, and it was one less thing to do. The nurses asked if I experienced phantom pain now that medicine wasn't getting in the way. It wasn't constant, but now and then phantom pain shot through me so hard and fast that my legs froze in its grip. Sometimes my sleep was interrupted by fingers of pain pressing on my invisible foot, squeezing and twisting. I could feel my 'toes' from big to pinky. Sometimes my 'feet' ached with cold. I warmed them by rubbing my calves and tricking my brain. My feet always felt like they were there, which was a key to walking.

Linda, my physiotherapist, told me that since my skin was severely compromised, learning to walk would take time. I appreciated how important it was to her that her clients walked well. Half-assing it was not her style.

"What about stairs?" I asked her, "How long will it be until I can do stairs?"

There were two sets of stairs in physiotherapy, one set smaller than the other. Even with the easy set of stairs I leaned heavily on the railing next to it to climb up one step. Stepping down was harder. I felt like I was on the edge of a cliff as I attempted to step down onto a stair in front of me, my legs wobbly, and one foot hovering in the air while the other tried to land, terrified at any moment that I could fall.

A year ago I had gone camping with a group of guy friends in the beautiful mountains of British Columbia. I swam in glacier fed lakes, hiked, and stood on cliff tops, enjoying the breathtaking views, and now I couldn't make my foot land on the stair in front of me.

I was told it takes strength, skill, and time to do stairs properly. I'd heard it all before, and began to take it personally, like time was out to get me. I was afraid too much time would pass by and apathy would set in. I had seen firsthand what it did to people, how they gave up and grew despondent. I couldn't let that be me.

Sensing my growing desperation, Linda took advantage of a quiet afternoon and wheeled me to a long sloped driveway around the back of the rehab center, and said, "One day you'll be ready to do this."

I drew a deep breath. "I hope so." Walking up and down this steep hill was like an able-bodied person climbing a mountain on a dare. I wanted to be positive, and knew that approach to this next stage of recovery could affect my outcome. I wanted to be a believer, to borrow Linda's vision and breathe life into my own.

When I was allowed, I walked indoors on shiny flat surfaces that were free of obstacles. Up and down, up and down, between parallel bars. I was always within reach of something or someone if I needed help. When I felt able, I walked around the center through corridors, to the elevators, to meals with a walker. Unlike the walker in the hospital, this one had wheels.

Roll the walker, step, roll, step. I felt so tall. The majority of people were in wheelchairs, and I was an Amazon among them.

Now, I had my eye on conquering a square piece of green land just outside G.F. Strong. On weekends, dads and kids played there, kicking or throwing balls back and forth. Spring wound its way through the park, in the green of the grass and the flowering of the trees. I couldn't help but be stirred by the hope that spring carried. Looking around, I wondered who lived in the charming weathered houses that stood around the park. There was something comforting about those long-established homes, like they had seen it all, done it all, and resolutely continued to stand and keep watch over the park and its visitors. The sidewalk running around the park beckoned to me.

In order to build up my endurance, I needed to be able to get around this park. Weather permitting, my plan was to be out there every day, walking.

It was a quiet day and I looked both ways. The big ticket items, like passing cars, were out of the way, now I needed to pay close attention to the small things—the things most of us take for granted.

Broken glass winked at me as I crossed the street.

A crack in the pavement loomed large to my right.

The small wheels of my walker hit some loose gravel, which forced me to stop, gather the wits that threatened to spill out of me, and try again. Slow and steady wins the race.

The sidewalk was just ahead.

I had to avoid the grass that lay next to it, nowhere near ready for that yet. Grass hid uneven ground, and I relied heavily on my eyesight for balance. If I couldn't see the shape of the ground, there was no way I could risk walking on it. I really didn't feel like having my face smashed into the ground, powerless to get up.

The sidewalk dipped down slightly, so I could push the walker along it and move my way up onto the sidewalk. My heart pounded a cadence against my jangling nerves. One misstep, and I would tip over...

A sigh of relief. Both feet planted firmly on the sidewalk. *I did it!* Concentrating, I looked down at my feet. Roll, step, roll, step down the sidewalk. I smiled. At no one. At everything. I was outside. I made it. And it felt good.

What struck me about walking was the absorption it took. It required not only physical strength, but all my brain power just to plant one foot in front of the other. If someone accompanied me for a walk, I often couldn't hold up my end of the conversation because I needed to focus. Talking was a distraction. Even listening proved to be difficult.

Sometimes Scott joined me for a walk, and if I grew quiet, he asked, "Are you tired?" I nodded. He'd respond, "Okay, I'll shut up, now." He knew I needed to concentrate.

There was a grocery store not far from rehab, and one of my goals on my to-do list for the disabled was to walk there, buy something, anything, and return home with it. One Friday night, I had a craving for Haagen Daaz chocolate chocolate chip ice cream and, dammit, I would get some.

I was about to embark on a field trip.

I rolled and stepped my way through rehab, rode the elevator down two floors and made my way out the front doors. Ten minutes later, I stood in the freezer section searching for my beloved ice cream.

There were small things that I took for granted when I wasn't, well, crippled. I hadn't given any thought to opening a door, so I never appreciated how you had to put some weight into pulling it. I wanted to get my ice cream off the shelf and into my greedy hands, but how was I going to keep my balance while opening the door, free up one of my hands from my death grip on the walker to grab the ice cream, then drop it into the basket without having the door bang back into place?

When I was in my wheelchair, living from a sitting position, I had similar issues about having to rethink and strategize everything.

I fumbled my way through, feeling my heart beat in my ears, wondering if other shoppers were staring at me as I hung onto anything that was within reach and stable. I hoped no one would help me. I wanted to do this alone.

Flushed and flustered I managed not to tip over, kept my heart from jumping out of my chest, and grabbed my ice cream. I shuffled over to the checkout and took my place in the line-up closest to me. As I stood in line and time ticked by, I quickly realized this was the toughest task. Not taking my first steps, not making my way around a park, and not attempting to open a door with ease. Standing still while waiting my turn was going to be my greatest feat.

I vaguely remembered Linda telling me how one must have stamina for this—to stand in one spot and rest all of your weight on these two artificial legs made to hold you up. It was trying on your body. Bilateral amputees use forty to fifty percent more energy than the average person. It hurt to stand in one spot, and I didn't expect that. I heard Linda's voice in the back of my mind. "Shift your weight from one foot to the other."

So I shifted. Back and forth, back and forth. I also leaned heavily on my walker. It helped, but my body lost patience.

Two more people to go...

Back and forth.

Finally. My turn.

The cashier smiled at me as she scanned my ice cream and put it in a bag. She asked if I had a membership card as I handed her my money.

What? "No, I don't."

"Would you like to have one? You can collect points and there are discounts. All you have to do is fill out your name and address."

I can't stand here a second longer. "No, no. I'm good." I smiled like I didn't have a care in the world. Like standing there filling out a form, which may as well have been a twenty page document, wouldn't cause me to fall over from sheer exhaustion. My legs prickled like they had awakened after falling asleep. I had to get out of there.

"Oh, okay. It only takes a sec."

"I really have to go, but thanks."

"Maybe next time then?"

The entire exchange took mere seconds, but to me, she was setting up camp for the night. In a high voice attempting enthusiasm, but bordering on shrill, I squeaked, "Sure, okay!"

She handed me my bag and I threw it into my basket.

Ten minutes later I entered my room.

I dropped the ice cream on the table next to my bed, beside the spoon I had kept from dinner in anticipation for this event—because it was an event. I pressed the button to lower the bed and eased myself onto it, then collapsed starfish-style across the mattress. I stripped down, peeled off my legs, which landed with a thud on the linoleum floor. I looked down at them splayed on the floor, one on top of the other, and sighed. I'd get to those later.

I got into pajamas and settled under the blankets. I picked up the remote to turn on the small TV in my room, flipped through channels until I found *X-Files*, and savored the first spoonful of slightly melted chocolate chocolate chip ice cream, cold and sweet, victory on my tongue.

19
Exposed

I looked around the table at faces I was just getting to know. It was one of the weekends I got to spend at home, and Scott and I were at a pub.

A girl sitting next to me spoke up eagerly. "Heidi, I was just thinking of you the other day."

"Oh?"

"I was in the shower shaving my legs and I thought 'Heidi is so lucky she doesn't have to do this anymore.' "

Quiet fell upon the table. It slammed into us. Everyone's smiles froze into Cheshire Cat grins. Forks clattered onto plates, and some of us hurriedly gulped down beer. All I could hear was the clink of glasses at the tables next to us and the exploding brain activity of people thinking *this did not just happen.*

"You're so lucky you don't have to worry about that anymore."

She wasn't kidding. And I had no retort.

She grinned, eyes wide and oblivious. I knew her name, but I didn't know her. She was a friend of a friend. A friend of a friend telling me how lucky I am that I don't have to shave my legs because they aren't here anymore.

All eyes were on me as I fished around for an answer. I mimicked the Cheshire Cat grin until someone found their voice and began to loudly ask questions of the person beside them, forcing the attention away from me. Color returned to our faces and function restored to our bodies.

I didn't know whether to be hurt or outraged. I wanted to laugh because this was funny. Awkward as hell, but hilarious. I didn't know what would possess a person to let those words come from her mouth.

Each time I went home, I was handed another piece of reality, another way in which my life had changed and my future carved in stone. I had more time to think here, maybe too much.

I should have died, but I was still here. How could I tell anyone that I wasn't grateful to be alive? I thought I should feel relieved, but I wasn't. Betty died. And I didn't.

I often thought about guests on talk shows telling their harrowing tales of how they came to survive and overcome tragedy. Tears were shed, and they were grateful just to be alive. All the while, the heads of the audience nodded along as they dabbed their eyes. I felt enormous expectation to have the appropriate responses for the people in my life. Like the heads in the audience, I wanted to have their heads bob along, satisfied with what I was saying.

When people asked how I felt, I was never sure of what the response should be. It depended on the day. I tried to tie up the end of those conversations with 'I'm thankful to be alive,' but, it didn't come out that way.

Some days I was *fine*. That was a good day. Fine sufficed. Other days, it was harder to find adequate words to describe what was going on with me. Devastation was a good word to use. It was strong, decisive. It fit the situation. What happened was devastating. But, more than that, I felt exposed.

In the hospital, it was about survival. I fought for my life and then recovered from each surgery. Every day was the same, and I was safe within my four walls. At G.F. Strong, reality sank in, and I had to face the fact that my life, as I knew it, had unraveled. I needed to regain my independence and work my way towards freedom. While I did venture outside, I was mostly in a fortress of routine and patients and accessibility for the handicapped. But it became harder to hide.

My body wore everything that had gone wrong, and evidence of the crash was all over me. I felt vulnerable having my pain on display. I was open to be stared at and pitied. By looking at me, you could see my devastation, and my grief was suddenly a friend's grief, a stranger's grief. Because people could see me, or had been introduced to me, they shared in it, recalling stories of people they knew who had suffered through trauma or a time when they used a wheelchair. Everyone could relate.

I listened, but I got tired of being a trigger for grief, and tired of people feeling like they knew me. I wanted to shout some days, "This isn't me!" There was more to me than my injuries. And there was desperation in me to make sure this proved to be true.

I was hesitant to talk about Betty, and rarely did. If she came up, there were more questions.

In rehab, or around town, my throat constricted and my eyes remained dry as I hurried through the part of the story where my friend died on impact. My reluctance to talk about her passing away, even with close friends, must have seemed odd to people. There was sacredness to my friend and her death, and I didn't want people to stick their fingers into it and stir it up. She deserved peace. With Angela and Loraleigh, I talked about the good things, the funny stories, her laugh, but I didn't like to talk about the end of Betty's life.

She died in that car. She died next to me in that car. And I was pried from that car, alive. I didn't know how to talk about that. I wanted to respect Betty's family and the loss of their sister and daughter. My back was straight and my face strong as people mourned her. I was her protector. It would be nearly two years before I let myself cry for Betty.

~~~

A local reporter came to my parents' house to interview me one of the weekends I came home. The story of the car accident had been followed closely in my home town, and he was there to follow up on my progress. There was more talk about the driver. Would he be charged? Would this be brought to trial?

I was angry that day. Angry that he was there, angry that he was intruding on something I didn't want to talk about, angry

I'd agreed to the interview. I didn't want to do it, but I thought it was the right thing to do. I was told people were interested and wanted to know how I was doing.

He asked me a number of questions. He asked me about my best friend, Betty. I bristled. "She wasn't my best friend." The words fell from my mouth, flat, before I could stop them.

He looked up from his pad of paper, surprised.

Wings of shame beat against me as butterflies lodged themselves in my stomach. I didn't know what I tried to accomplish when I said that. Of course, she was one of my best friends. Of course, I loved her like a sister. That's how I introduced her to people, as the sister I never had.

But all I wanted was for him to go away. I wanted for all of this to go away. I wanted Betty's family to have some peace, and maybe I wanted to have the sensationally sad story of two best friends in a horrific car crash to change. If I dropped the 'best' from it, maybe it would lessen the blow, somehow. Maybe the reporter would leave her out of the story altogether, so her family wouldn't have to see Betty's name in print and be reminded, as if they weren't reminded every day, that she wasn't here anymore. It was ridiculous, really. There was nothing I could do to change what had happened, and now I was coming across as some selfish, sullen victim.

I wondered if the survivors being interviewed on talk shows were doing their best to meet expectations, or were they shell-shocked like me and drew upon interviews before them, citing the correct answers. "Yes, I look at life differently now. I am grateful. The world has opened up, and I no longer take anything for granted."

I couldn't wait for the day when I took things for granted again. I couldn't jump out of bed, or climb out lazily if I wanted to. As soon as it was time to get out of bed, it was with purpose, which entailed grabbing my liners, sliding them on to my stubby legs, sticking them into fake ones, and then pulling and tugging on the gel sleeves, which held my legs in place.

My showers were drastically altered as well. I showered on a bench, using my arms and hands for balance. It took a while to feel secure, precariously perched on a bench, slippery with water and soap. Heading to a destination that I hadn't been to before unnerved me. Would there be stairs? If there were, was there a railing to hold onto? Would I be able to squeeze my wheelchair into the washroom? Would I hold people up behind me when I stepped onto the stairs? I moved so slowly.

Everything was painstakingly considered, with my brain working as hard as my body. Even turning over in my bed was something to adapt to. It took effort to shift my body until I found a comfortable spot. Feet, I discovered, weren't only for walking or running. It was all the little things I missed so much. One of my favorite positions to sit in was cross-legged or curling my feet under me. I would never be able to sit like that again.

As I got out more, I tucked two collapsible canes in between the cushion and the arm of my chair. A walker was harder to transport, especially if I had to use my chair. Even though I was unsteady on canes, they were the easiest aids to bring. I went to a book store, one of my favorite things to do, searching for that perfect book, when I realized I couldn't squat down to look at the books on the lowest shelf. I stood in the aisle, leaning on my canes, overcome with loss.

When I returned to rehab, I asked Linda, "Will I ever be able to squat, the kind of squat where you're down on your haunches? Is that something I could develop over time?" But, I already knew the answer.

I didn't have ankles or the balls of my feet to roll onto, and prosthetic legs that come to the knee don't bend. I hoped for a different answer.

Linda was straightforward, "You'll never be able to do that."

No books on the bottom shelf. No food, no items of clothing. Bent and straining, everything on the bottom shelf would always be just beyond my reach. I relied upon her candor, and appreciated her no bullshit approach to life. I just couldn't stomach it that day. I left physiotherapy early to nurse my anger.

While I sometimes lied to keep peace, I never lied to myself. I had enough going on without faking my feelings. If I was angry, I allowed it to take up some space inside me, giving it room to vent.

Perhaps a way to keep honest was to journal. It was suggested often as a way to dissect and sort my grief. I kept journals growing up, wrote poetry, even tried my hand at a novel. If I did this, I'd have to stare at grief on a page, in print. I'd move my hand up and down writing about my feelings.

I liked journals, hard cover journals opening to fresh pages. New journals were a clean slate, a fresh beginning. I started my journals with the intent of keeping them neat and tidy, but eventually my hand had to catch up to my brain, and moved so fast I could barely read my writing.

I didn't want to spoil a brand new journal with heartache, with tears and confusion. For this first stab at writing, I found a loose piece of paper at the nurse's station and sprawled out on my rehab bed. I held a pen, my hand poised over the paper, waiting for words to find me.

Time ticked by and finally I wrote, 'I don't know what to say.' Followed by a profound, '...'

Just then there was a knock at my door. I wasn't expecting company, so when an unfamiliar female face greeted me, I assumed it was a new staff member.

"Hi, Heidi. I just wanted to stop by and say hello."

"Hi." I sat up in my bed.

"I don't know if you know me. I knew Betty."

"Oh."

"How are you? I've been, we've all been, praying for you."

"I'm okay," I said warily. "Thank you."

After some small talk about the routine of rehab, she took a few tentative steps into the room. "I was wondering if you had ever considered sharing your story, or writing it down. It's an incredible story I'm sure many people would love to hear. Need to hear."

I was curt. "No, I haven't thought about it." I couldn't even put my thoughts on a piece of paper.

"Well, if you couldn't write it, maybe I could help you with that. We could turn your story into a book." She tucked her hair behind her ear and smiled.

"No, I don't think so. But thanks."

"Okay, well, you might change your mind." She turned to leave. "Bye, Heidi. It was nice to see you."

"Bye."

I didn't know what to make of that. I should have invited her to sit down, I should have told her it was nice meeting her, too. But as soon as she started talking about a book, cordiality left me. I didn't know if I would ever write a book, and it was far too soon to tell, but I certainly wasn't going to have a stranger write it, even a well-meaning stranger.

I folded the mostly blank piece of paper into tiny squares and slid it into my nightstand drawer.

20
Season of Scars

Eleven months had passed since the crash, and summer was approaching. Girls my age with shiny hair, exposed skin, and polished toes, flipped their hair and complained about the heat, while I was sucker-punched in the gut. I couldn't believe I'd never know this again. I was breathless with memories, suffocated by the sun.

Before the crash, summer was my favorite season, filled with hours at the lake, reading until the words blurred together, adjusting my bathing suit straps for minimal tan lines. My year began in the fall, not in January. Summer was my chance to shed the worries and mistakes of the past year and live carefree for a few months until I got to start over.

In the wake of June 12, 1998, the summer was cruel to me, a joke. I couldn't do what I wanted. I couldn't wear what I wanted to wear.

At the edge of the beach, near the runners and cyclists, I sat on a wooden bench. Scott and I decided to leave rehab and spend some time outside on one of the first hot days of the year in May. I had walked from the car to the bench, leaning my canes against the arm of the bench. He asked, "Do you want a drink?"

"I would love a drink. Do you mind getting it? I think it's going to be too much work to walk over today."

"Sure." It wasn't long before Scott was a speck on the pathway as he went in search of cold drinks. I couldn't walk on sand, the tiny grains shifting and sliding under me would have made it impossible to balance. A safe distance from the beach, I observed the hot day's participants, protected by the shade of a tree. Hiding behind my dark sunglasses, I was assaulted by the sounds and smells of summer.

My ears tuned in to the slap slapping of flip-flops, my nose picked up the unmistakable essence of Coppertone as it wafted over in air thick with heat, making me nostalgic. All I could feel and breathe were scars so red and legs encased in silicone, plastic, and metal, along with skin that stretched too tight and itched all the time. I scratched until I bled. The sun was my enemy, and I was consumed by Never. Never ever, never more, never again.

Summer played like a favorite movie. There I am hitching up my jeans as I wade into the ocean, blissful as the ice cold water runs over my feet, the churn of the water as I kick, kick my way through. Squealing children splashing each other. Bikinis! Shorts! Fun flirty sundresses!

I was an outsider, a voyeur. I tried to swap these stories, this montage, with less vivid pictures, muted colors, and the volume turned down. Instead, my feet won't be scraped by the rocks anymore. I'll have less chance of getting skin cancer now. Less clothes to choose from, therefore saving me money!

It didn't work.

I tore my eyes away from the beach and focused on the cement pathway in front of me, hoping for something less traumatic. No such luck. The pathway teemed with legs. Legs pumping, cycling, gliding. Feet flying, skipping, hurrying.

I mourned my body, nauseous with what wasn't mine. I shut my eyes. But open or shut, all I could see were bare feet and smooth skin. My skin prickled with heat, with exhaustion, and envy.

I noticed people's stares, their sidelong glances. Aiming for discreet, their eyes slid from my arms to my canes before turning away in haste so they wouldn't get caught. Children couldn't tear their eyes from me until a parent grabbed their hand and tugged them away.

While I could go outside and sit on a bench, or walk around in the sunshine, summer was no longer a symbol of freedom. I recalled Christmas and the realization of my firsts, a year of unwanted new beginnings. My first major surgery, my first steps with prosthetic legs, the first time I lost a friend, and now the first summer. My heart twisting, I stared straight ahead. I could get through today and tomorrow, but what about next year? I would face this season again. I looked down at the pressure garments on my arms starting where my t-shirt sleeves ended. I was constricted by the pressure garments underneath my clothes, the elastic digging into my flesh. Hidden under the garments was an ever present colostomy bag. Forget fashionable pants. Mine were thin wide pants so they fit over my bulky legs. I brought my hands to my heart. Beneath my hands, under good skin, I measured each beat. Summer was over before it began.

I would have to adjust and that became my life—a series of adjustments.

I wouldn't be lying on a bright worn beach towel, the sun hot, coloring my skin. I wouldn't dip my toes into the calm and cool of a lake. I wouldn't get sand stuck between my toes, gritty and hot while walking along the edge of the ocean.

One day, I knew I would stand at the shoreline and admire the ocean's vastness. I'd close my eyes and inhale the saltwater scent, feeling small in a big world. I would skim my hand along the top of the ocean and remember my days of contentment lying beside it, then swimming in it, sleepy with sun and fresh air. I would appreciate summer's beauties from a distance, with keen observation. I couldn't be in it the way I once was.

But for now, I wanted to rush through the hot season, to sprint ahead and get it over with, so I could look for the leaves to change color and meet cooler temperatures. Grafted skin cut off sweat glands, so once I became hot, I simmered because my body had lost its natural efficiency to cool. It was easier to be sick in the winter, a perfect environment of gray and bare. Summer shed light on all that had gone wrong, making my loss more obvious. Summer was where I was born again to a stripped and mangled body.

I looked for Scott, anxious to be rescued from my thoughts, and spotted him walking toward me, drinks in his hands. I wanted to lose myself in conversation, in him, and forget about summer.

He held up two cups. "I found some lemonade."

I took a long sip from the straw. "Thanks, I needed this." I looked over at him. "I'm happy you're back. It's hard to be here."

I braced myself for a pep talk. A few times, he had advised me to accept strangers' curiosity and my changes, telling me it was okay that I'm different. I felt this push to move forward, and on more than one occasion, I told him I don't want to be different. I'll move forward, but not today.

"I know." He covered my hand with his.

I smiled, relieved. He knew me.

21

The Girl From the Car Accident

I still looked sick eleven months later. I knew I looked sick. All that was missing was a hospital gown and a nurse with a ready needle to push medication through an IV.

I stuck out, but I held my back straight and kept my head up. I was shopping with my mom at a mall in the city. We'd called it a day when she decided to pop into one more store. I parked my wheelchair next to the pretzel stand near the entrance of the food court in a vain attempt to blend in with the crowd.

I noticed a tall blonde man a few feet away from me. He looked to be in his late twenties or early thirties and had that put-together look; well dressed and clean shaven. He caught my eye and approached me.

Please don't talk to me. Please don't look meaningfully into my eyes, say you're going to pray for me, or ask me what happened. Please go the other way. Please just ask me where Club Monaco is.

The tall blonde man stopped at the arm of my chair. He said, "I just wanted to tell you that you're beautiful." He said it without pity. He just held it out to me, like a promise.

He turned and left. I whispered a soft, "Thank you," but I don't know that he heard me.

His words were an unexpected benediction, reaching out and cradling my face. An answer to a prayer I hadn't thought to utter.

I treasured those moments of grace that found their way to me at odd times, when I wasn't looking, catching me off guard, and piercing my gnawing emptiness. Sneak attack was the best way to get to me.

I didn't tell my mom when she returned. I kept it to myself like a child hoarding secrets, afraid the spell would be ruined with one touch, one word, and it would disappear in a puff of smoke.

It came to me later, in the days and months to follow, that every person needs to feel beautiful, especially when we are at our worst, our ugliest. To have someone reach beneath the surface, past the scars, and see you. To recognize you are a marvel, you are something to behold. To honor your strengths before your weaknesses. To acknowledge how hard you try.

I thought about kind words and actions stirring life in parched and forgotten places, and how I was starving when a stranger happened to stop to feed me. For a few seconds my life felt magical, like God's intervention, at a time where there was little to believe in.

~~~

A week after my strangely wonderful encounter, Scott and I sat on the couch in the basement of my parents' home, having another day off from rehab. I shivered, not from cold, but from the emptiness that was present at every turn, reminding me of my hard-earned existence and my aloneness in it. I whispered to Scott, to anyone, anything, "Does it ever get better?"

Scott was quiet for a moment. "I think it's going to be love that will get you through."

I didn't know what I was looking for. I just wanted the hole in me to disappear. I had love, but what would love *do?* Love wasn't good enough. Love mocked in its inadequacy.

I looked at him, confused. "Love?"

"Love."

How could he be so sure? I felt bottomless in my need. Nothing could fill me up. Love would sink like a stone and be lost.

And what kind of love? Scott's love? My family's? God's love? I had heard about God's love all my life. *God's love never fails. God loves everyone. God is love.* God came up a lot.

I grew up going to church and then made my own choices about God. My brothers and I were asked to attend church with my parents until we turned twelve. After that, we had permission to decide whether we wanted to keep going or not. My younger brothers' church-going petered out in their teens, but I continued going to church and began to shape my own thoughts about faith while I sat in the pews.

I saw God as big, loving, and compassionate. As a child I thought God could do anything—He could swoop down from the sky and take me flying. Me and God on a magic carpet ride soaring through the air. I used to look for Him in the clouds and write notes, hoping He'd retrieve them when I left them by some shrubs near my house. I believed in a magical and mysterious God, a God with tricks up His long sleeves, meant to delight.

I was also taught that God knows everything, sees everything. Always present. Sometimes that brought assurance and, at other times, guilt when I couldn't escape under His roving eye. I got older, and some of the magic and fear disappeared, but the mystery of God and the universe surrounding us, the bigness of God, was still there for me. I didn't have all the answers, and didn't pretend otherwise. I was content to stay in the mystery.

Love and God was supposed to save me. That's what the Bible says. That's what the Church believed. I wasn't so sure.

If God is so great, couldn't He make me better? Where were the tricks? Where was the magic? Where was love?

I knew no one was granted immunity from bad things happening. Bad things happened all the time around the world. Nothing would be gained by me shaking my fist at the sky, demanding, "Why me?" Because, why anyone? I lived in an imperfect world.

People made choices, some good, and some bad. I didn't think this was about God as much as someone who made a choice to drive recklessly, making Betty and me unwitting targets.

Being a Christian was complicated, especially when things went wrong. It can't make up its mind, and is riddled with conflicting messages. My faith should increase with each passing day, yet Thomas doubted. I could find comfort in Jesus crying out in the Garden of Gethsemane, begging His Father to take death from

Him. I should be angry because I must be, and it's okay to be angry. Even the Psalmists were angry.

Anything good that happened was hailed as God's work. I didn't agree. *I* was doing the work. God wasn't going to surgery every day, stretched out and strapped down for hours while doctors worked over Him, painstakingly putting Him back together. That was me.

It was said that God was with me. When I saw God, it was in my nurses' hands, in the talents and skills of my doctors, and in the hope and compassion that family and friends brought with them when they came to see me.

So I was confused by Scott's proclamation that love would heal me. "What do you mean?"

"Heidi, we'll do this a day at a time, and I think love is a big part of that."

"*I* am doing this. *I'm* getting through it. It's just that..." I stopped.

"It's just that what?"

"I want to feel better, and I can't. I don't. I'm trying so hard. But all I feel is lost. I keep thinking it could be worse, like that's supposed to comfort me. And sometimes I'm just so angry. I'm so angry this is my life."

My voice dropped to a whisper, "I don't have my legs, Scott. My *legs*. My body is..." I used my hands as punctuation, waving them around to make my point until they fell to my side, defeated.

We were silent, my words and our sorrow planted themselves between us. I couldn't be fixed, and I would have given anything to be fixed. I was stripped of what I knew, down to the bare bones of myself. Could I be capable? Am I enough?

From that moment in ICU, when Scott asked if I wanted to live, I was confronted with choices, life and death choices. When I moved from immediate danger to recovery, I was confronted with *how* I was going to do this. Would I be a victim or a survivor?

When people told me that everything happens for a reason, I wanted to laugh. What possible reasons could there be for mothers and fathers to lose their sons or daughters? What reason was there when a limb was taken, a body charred, a life turned inside out? I looked everywhere, examined my life, and still couldn't come up with a reason.

I didn't want to waste time on clichés. I couldn't search for deeper truths others had found. I wouldn't live someone else's journey. I wanted to find my own truths and make my own way. Not only did I want love to save me, I wanted it to set me free.

Daily, I encountered people consumed by the tragedy and not by the fight. I'd witnessed people getting by, existing, and shutting down. Their identities became wrapped up in what happened rather than 'who they are.' Overnight, I was a different person, and this wasn't the plan for my life, my dreams, to go up in smoke.

I was now Heidi, the girl from the car accident. I acquired labels and titles I didn't want. Amputee and burn survivor weren't titles I wore proudly. I should have been proud. I was encouraged to be proud. But I wanted to simply be Heidi.

Recovery dominated my life. Each day became about getting through. My legs and skin were in front of me, demanding my attention. I was told it gets better. I was told that one day it wouldn't be like this. I hoped it was true. God, I hoped it was true. In the meantime, my plight wasn't changing. Physically, I was at the mercy of my body. But emotionally, my questions and the answers I came up with were vital to how I finished.

I knew this: Fire hadn't destroyed who I was. I belonged to me as much as I belonged to God. I would rise above, not as some glorious phoenix from the ashes, but living one day at a time, piecing myself back together. Could I emerge scathed and scarred, and meet my definition of whole?

22

A New Ordinary

I stared at pages of multiple choice feelings, questions leading me to answer if I was depressed or not, sane or insane. Could I sleep, did I have nightmares, anxious thoughts, was I obsessive in my thoughts or actions, and did I feel as though the world was out to get me? In the waiting room of my new psychiatrist's office, I filled in the small empty circles meant to define me.

It was early June, nearing the one year anniversary of the crash. I had been at G.F. Strong for five months, and my team of people had been preparing for me to go, and this time I was ready.

My social worker found me a place to live, a co-op apartment in False Creek near Granville Island, steps away from the ocean. When my mom, Scott, and I climbed out of the car, I had to shield my eyes from the bright sun glinting off the ocean. I was giddy as I took the ramp that led down to the entrance of the building. "Wheee!" I took my hands off the wheels and rolled, hands in the air, like a kid, toward the glass door.

We buzzed our way into the building and were let in to the apartment by a woman on the co-op board who ran the place. Tall and slender with short and curly black hair, the woman was chatty and bright as she showed us around the building. It was bare bones and cheerless with its narrow kitchen, white walls, and thin blue carpet, but it was on the bottom floor, wheelchair-accessible, and mine for the time-being. It was perfect.

I was moving to a coveted area of Vancouver, and I was thrilled. I would be on my own, having to rely on myself to get things done. Physiotherapy would be on an outpatient basis, and this was the closest to normal I'd felt in a year.

Between the things I brought from G.F. Strong and bought from Ikea, I could now call my apartment home.

Now that I was settled, it was time to listen to my lawyer. Nearly a year had passed, and the driver of the other vehicle was still under investigation and hadn't been charged yet because there was confusion over who was driving.

Two brothers, ages 17 and 19, were in the car and claimed it was the 17 year old, the minor, driving. After their car hit mine, neighbors spilled out of their homes and people pulled over to focus on Betty and me, who were trapped inside my burning car. No one saw who was the passenger or driver. They didn't notice them getting out of the car, or whether the brothers were hurriedly forming a plan.

When a police officer asked about the driver, the 17 year old stepped forward to shoulder the blame. Within a week, the police received an anonymous tip that it was the other way around, that Jeff, the 19 year old, was the driver. They lied to protect Jeff, who had been prohibited from driving, yet drove anyway.

I'd heard Jeff had a record of bad driving, and this was another strike, the biggest strike. This time he had gone too far, killing Betty, and causing me to suffer major burns and multiple amputations. I needed to keep the facts of the ongoing investigation far away from me so I could concentrate on healing. I knew there was a lot going on behind the scenes. My parents fought hard for justice, and a detective was brought onto the case.

Whenever Jeff was brought up, I wanted to clamp my hands over my ears and turn the other way. I never asked questions. I didn't want to know because I already knew too much. I knew the boys sat on the curb and called us bitches for getting in the way. I knew they stuck to their lie while we were engulfed in flames. I couldn't let their depraved cruelty creep in. I did not want to waste time being angry, fixating on Jeff. How damaged must a person be to feel that way, to lash out like that?

I had to take one thing at a time.

I knew we had to deal with the insurance company at this point. If this crash turned into a criminal matter, it wouldn't affect the settlement. Either way, there would be compensation for me. Giving the driver my time interfered with my recovery. He had done enough, and his choices affected my every day. I refused to give him more power in my life, to let him hurt me more than I'd been hurt.

Counseling was part of the agreement for an upcoming settlement that my lawyer and insurance company agreed upon. I had to go to counseling to get diagnosed. Was I a wreck? How much damage had been done, and what dollar amount could be put to it? I didn't understand how the process of settlement worked, how they formulated their decisions. I just did what I was told.

Did I answer the questions according to how I felt pre-accident, or was it how I felt now, today, post-accident? I was advised to answer honestly and fill in the one that best suited me on questions whose answers were vague.

I wanted to appear normal, although I'd have to be a psychopath to not feel all kinds of different emotions after a car slammed into me. I wanted to be fine, but not too fine, and keep my feelings somewhere in the middle. It was a case of "When in doubt choose C." I aimed for a little depressed with a hint of optimism. I felt safest there. I wasn't likely to have people searching my house for an alarming number of pills or a gun, and I wouldn't come across as numb to the point of needing psychiatric care. I realized how strange it was to still care what people thought of me. I had gone through serious trauma, and I worried I'd be perceived as depressed!

I didn't make for a receptive counseling patient. I was a good patient in the hospital, but the last thing I wanted was to be in the hands of yet another doctor, another person who didn't know me. There was nothing I wanted to talk about that I hadn't already discussed with Scott and close friends. I met with the psychiatrist twice. I assumed I had passed my depression test when he didn't give me a prescription before handing me over to a counselor on his team for the following appointment.

I wasn't very forthcoming in my sessions with the counselor, either. She put her clipboard down and looked at me. "This isn't going to work if you won't talk to me."

I stared at her hands folded in her lap. I was caught. "I don't know what to say. I'm just getting through it as best as I can." I fell back on my hospital 'things will work out' mantra.

"You need to trust me. I'm here to listen, and I'm here to help."

She was frustrated. I understood that. I was frustrated, too. Even though nearly a year had passed, I was still reeling from what had happened. After all this time, I didn't know how to make sense of it, let alone sift through it with a stranger. Yes, time had passed since the crash, but I was still so close to it I couldn't untangle me from the day, yet. I hoped time would soften me, but there were still so many feelings, that I found it nearly impossible to feel.

I was in counseling because it was required. Everything I said would be checked and underlined by my lawyer and the insurance company. When I first arrived at the office, I signed a contract giving them permission to scrutinize my feelings.

She meant well, but the client-counselor relationship was doomed. While I could have benefited from her expertise, I couldn't be myself with her. I found it hard not to feel like I was being interviewed, and my instinct was to put on my best face and biggest smile. What could she possibly say to me that would make this better? What helpful tips and advice could she give me other than to tell me this is my life now and I must deal with it?

Betty was gone. I was in a wheelchair. Please don't make me go over the heartbreaking details and my disfigurement. I fought hard not to give in to the tragedy of the grotesque, the hideous underneath my clothing. Stating the truth, the obvious, wouldn't change anything.

I had to talk, so I talked. Not about the car crash or my injuries, and not about loss, but about everything else — my family, my childhood, my previous life. I was indifferent to what transpired in the office. What happened outside of it was another matter entirely. Real life existed there. I had been cut open and sewn together for months, and now with every appointment, I grew sick, sick of being dissected. Sick of being laid bare and exposed. I needed a break from being in clinical sterile settings in the attempt to make me better. I needed out.

I was also sent to vocational counseling to, again, determine my worth. What kind of job could I have been capable of if I wasn't injured? My intelligence was tested to determine my future, and covered math, science, and English. More multiple choice, more small circles. If I was dumb, the outcome wouldn't be as great. *See, she wouldn't have made it in life anyway, so we don't have to pay her quite as much as we thought.*

My lawyer's job was to protect me and my future. It was protocol to send me to various places and appointments to be thorough. I paid him to go to bat for me with the insurance company. I had only met with my lawyer a few times and decided I liked him. He didn't use platitudes, and he was straightforward with me. He did his job.

Not every day was emotional, grueling work. I shopped for produce at the market and acquired small items at the corner store. I wheeled over to the neighborhood Starbucks nearly every day and bought lattes, sticking the coffee between my knees, while I rolled along the sun-dappled paths behind the apartments. I smiled and said hello to neighbors.

On one of my appointment days, I left my wheelchair and decided to walk home. I was still unable to walk as much as I wanted, but I decided to take the Handydart, the bus for the handicapped, to counseling, and I would return home by legs. It was downhill all the way home.

Before the crash, I was in the habit of running at midnight. If I couldn't sleep, I laced up my shoes and headed out into the cool night air. My head cleared as soon as my feet met the pavement. It was stupid to run at that late hour, but I loved the quiet at that time of night, the black of it, along with the few red lights to wait for. I missed it terribly. I lamented the ease of my body. I was light on my feet, restless, and a fidgeter.

My mind pulled in every direction when I knew what I wanted to do, what I used to do, but could no longer do. There was an uneven armistice between my head and body. My head was light and quick, but my body was heavy and unsure.

Changing my gait, toes straight ahead, made me feel unlike me. Walking was very deliberate, planned, and I had to remember to roll from heel to toe, careful not to make sudden movements. Even turning my head quickly could cause me to lose my balance. People shoving past me, innocent hurried movements, made me stumble, and I would have to stop and try again.

Leaving my walker behind at rehab, I had officially graduated from walker to canes. I still used my chair since I tired easily, but I used canes wherever possible. My canes were the nicest the medical supply store had — black aluminum with a small handle at the top, no old-person cane for me.

All of the rest I'd forced upon myself paid off. The wound on my right knee began to heal. The skin met in the middle, and the quarter-sized circle became a dime-sized circle, until it closed and was nothing more than a red dime-sized scar. Finally, time came around to my side and, combined with my hell-bent attitude, I became a better walker.

I stood outside the glass doors and visualized my route home. I considered which path would have fewer obstacles and less traffic lights. I walked to the end of the block, waited for the WALK signal, and crossed one of the busiest streets in Vancouver.

Deliberate and slow, I walked downhill. I had to be sure of each step and the placement of my foot, so as not to stumble and go flying down the hill. I didn't have the luxury of ankles to temper my steps, so my knees and hamstrings bore the brunt of the walk. I used my canes for balance, and they made a reassuring click each time I took a step.

I loved sunny days after it rained and the smell of the sun warming the earth. Today was one of those days. Walking of my own will and strength, I was finely tuned to the ground beneath my feet. I often needed to stop and rest, but today I wanted to try to get home without stopping. It felt good to push my body by stretching it to its limits like I used to when I ran.

It was days away from summer and in that half an hour it took to walk home, everything was all right with the world. It was glorious. Hard work, and glorious.

I let myself into my place and slumped against the door. I did it! I made it! Without stopping. I was on a runner's high. In that moment, I grasped how weary I'd grown from having my life revolve around appointments. Ready or not, I wanted to end all of it and live again.

Within weeks, I stopped physiotherapy. I was allowed to quit counseling, apparently the lawyers had all they needed. My life would be happening outside now. I lived in the city. Not at the hospital, not at rehab. No nurses. No safety net. Just me. I wanted to be completely, wholly here.

~~~

When people asked what I did for exercise now that I could no longer run, I pointed to my legs and my arms. Wheeling myself almost everywhere had given me strong muscular arms, and being an amputee was exercise enough, since I used up more energy than the average person.

Returning to running was never an option for me. There were other bilateral below-knee amputees out there who could, but my skin, or the lack of, wouldn't allow for me to run. As my mind got stronger, it outran my body. All the energy I'd had returned to my brain, and my legs couldn't keep up. I wanted to get out more, so I wheeled when I couldn't walk, and my arms and wheels became my legs.

I grew adept at maneuvering my chair up and down hills, squeezing through narrow doorways, and running errands. I lived in an area called False Creek that got very busy over the weekends. I was minutes away from Granville Island, a bit of a tourist hot spot, so I tried to avoid doing errands on Saturdays and Sundays, but once in a while boredom, visitors, or sun drove me out.

One weekend I passed by a few homeless men who had set up camp, their hats out, collecting money. My right knee ached that day, so my leg was propped up and stuck straight out in front of me. My left leg was encased in the prosthetic and bent at the knee like it should, with my foot resting on the footrest. One of the men lunged at me and grabbed the chair's handles, ready to push.

"Oh my God, Oh my God! What happened to you? You look worse than I do." He was sunburnt and unshaven, his clothes gray with age and wear.

I gripped the wheels and stopped him. "I'm okay." I smiled. "Really, I'm okay. I can do this myself. I do it almost every day."

"Oh, oh. Are you sure?"

I smiled and nodded, reassuring him of my competence.

He let go of my chair and shook his head, marveling at my misfortune as I made my way over the boardwalk.

I understood people wanted to help, but I didn't like strangers helping me without asking. My chair, at that point, was a part of me. People needed to ask if they wanted to push. Most people were gracious, opening doors for me, or parting like the Red Sea when I navigated my chair through a tight space, looking me in the eye when I asked a question or paid for my purchases. I was grateful they chose not to ask prying question because I really wanted to be treated, or ignored, like everyone else.

Being disabled could be a nuisance. Aside from the obvious, like the sadness that came with it, being disabled was a pain in the ass and it forced me to be a strategic thinker because I was re-entering my world in a different body

If I decided to walk, there was the possibility of a line-up somewhere. Waiting was exhausting. There were lines at the grocery store, the movie theatre, waiting to get into a dressing room to try on clothes. I knew I could take the wheelchair, but I so badly wanted to use my legs. If I walked for a few blocks, I scouted out places to sit along the way, since my legs tired quickly, and they swelled and prickled until I got out of them or got off of them. Low ledges on windows, benches, and steps made good pit stops.

Determined to be like everyone else, I didn't wave my big ol' handicapped flag to gain privileges, but once in a while I caved and surrendered to the fact that I was limited and needed help. It had its advantages. I had a handicapped parking pass, so I became everyone's favorite shopping partner. I could find a spot close to the mall, hang up my placard and walk or wheel the short distance to the door. My friends treated it like winning the lottery. "Yesss. Handicapped parking!"

I found that the more I got out, the better I felt. And the more I walked, the more *whole* I felt. People noticed me less, and I inched toward the anonymity I craved. I moved closer to ordinary.

23
Surfacing

I looked up at the tall building I was about to enter. Inside was the office of the doctor who would deliver news as to whether I could have the surgery to reroute my intestine and restore order, or if I was forever destined for the colostomy bag, something I loathed. I didn't want this attached to me for the rest of my life. It was necessary at the time because the burns to my backside were so deep, but I hoped I had healed enough to make this a distant memory.

Deep breath. Fingers crossed. And sending all my good thoughts into the universe, I felt my chances were good.

The doctor slid the chair by his desk over to make room for me. I rolled in and waited for him to speak. "Heidi, good news..."

I didn't hear anything after "good news." The stars were aligned. This would be my twentieth surgery, and this was the one I was most excited about. He proceeded to list what I should do pre-surgery, and I nodded as if I understood, but I lost focus. My mind was alight with the fact that this surgery was a wrong being made right, a small redemption. An undoing.

Alone in the elevator, I shimmied a jig in my wheelchair and belted out a quick squeal of joy. The sun was shining just for me as I got into the elevator and made my way down each floor to the lobby.

My surgery would take place at Vancouver General Hospital. When I left over a year ago, I was wheeled out and loaded onto a bus. This time, I walked in with my canes and was instantly struck by familiar smells and sounds. The hissing espresso machine, the cool recycled air, even doctors in scrubs were the same. But I felt different, bolder. I identified with the busy, bustling people rather than the patients in wheelchairs or walking their IV's. I was healthy.

I wondered if I'd go post-traumatic-stress-disorder upon entering the doors or, at the least, vibrate a little, but I didn't. Oddly, it felt safe, a little like coming home in a twisted, bizzaro way. I didn't relish becoming a patient again, even if only for a few days, but I knew I was in capable hands here, and this was a surgery I'd been looking forward to.

The surgery went well, and I would stay for the next few days to make sure my bowels recovered. On a strict, liquids-only diet, I thought I'd go crazy. After surgery and after vomiting from the anesthetic, I was hungry. It was going to be a long five days.

While my mom was visiting, she pulled a letter out of her purse. "I found this in our mailbox yesterday. It's from Lily."

I could see from the arch of her eyebrow she was surprised. I hadn't seen or heard from Lily since her awkward visit at Christmas.

"She *mailed* me a letter?" I sighed. "You have got to be kidding me. We live in the same town."

My mom shrugged. "Are you going to read it?"

"Maybe later."

I waited to open it after my parents left. Her letter was a list of how the past year had been hard on her. She went on to say that we were growing apart before the crash happened. At the hospital, she noticed there were people who did a better job of looking after me than she could. In summation, it had been a tough year for *her*.

I held the letter in my hands for a while, looking at the loops of her writing, the tidiness and the familiarity of it. I had been reading notes in her handwriting since I was fourteen.

Both of us liked to exercise, so our friendship was mostly spent outside going for walks, catching up on what was going on. We had been to Hawaii not long ago, just the two of us sunning ourselves at the beach and shopping in Waikiki. We had been in each other's lives for a long time.

Peace was her mission, but I didn't feel peaceful while folding the letter. To me it was a list of justifications, a plea for absolution, and an invitation for me to *call* or *write back.*

I lay still, my head on the pillow and concentrated on breathing. *She wrote me a letter.* My hands shook as I put her words aside. Lily's withdrawal. I couldn't fathom her unwillingness to walk through something so hard and so painful in my life.

The next day, friends came to visit and wheeled me down to the hospital café. I looked at their faces over our cups of coffee and recognized how rich I was in friendship, how loved and lucky I was to have these people in my life. It was a glaring distinction from Lily.

I wished Lily had never sent the letter, and I couldn't help but remain mystified at her claim of a "tough year." Out of our shared history and long-time friendship, I wanted to be fair; maybe it had been a hard year for her. I put myself in her shoes and turned the scenario over. *Would I have been there for her? What would I have done if she was in that bed?*

Angry, I felt my *tough year* trumped hers. We could have been there for each other. Hurt and spent, I didn't want the remainder of my stay to be about Lily, so I focused on being a good patient and the mundane, like when I could eat again. I looked forward to my first piece of toast.

A few days later I returned home with the letter and without a colostomy bag.

~~~

As I got better at using my legs and began picking up my life again, I decided I wanted my driver's license back. This was something I needed. With so much that was new and unwanted I was after another piece of my past and independence.

I went to Abbotsford one weekend to visit with family and asked my brother, Rick, if I could borrow his car. I lowered myself into the car, sliding in awkwardly to the driver's seat, and wrapped my hands around the steering wheel. I didn't start the car. I wanted to get used to being in one again and find the pedals with my fake feet. Surprised at how easy it felt, back and forth, I switched my foot from the accelerator to the brake until I knew how far apart they were and where to place my foot.

It was like coming home.

I turned on the ignition and pumped my leg to move my foot. After figuring out how much pressure to apply to the brake and accelerator, I drove slowly around my parents' neighborhood. I needed to drive out the memory of the old.

When I turned sixteen, I wasn't in a hurry to get my driver's license because I was nervous to get behind the wheel. At seventeen, my parents decided they were tired of driving me everywhere, and paid for lessons. As I grew comfortable being in the driver's seat, I fell in love with my newfound independence. It offered me freedom. Now I was reasserting my freedom all over again.

I had to re-do the driving test to prove I could handle a car with prosthetic legs, so any time I came home to Abbotsford, I drove as much as I could. The more I drove, the closer I got to the old me, and discovered how much I missed her. I fell in love again, and each trip brought me closer to independence, to spontaneity, and freedom...to the girl who enjoyed herself, who relished time alone in the car with the music playing loudly.

On one of those weekends in Abbotsford, I had time alone in the car, and my thoughts turned to Lily. Weeks after receiving her letter and still recovering from surgery, I decided to contact her. With my heart in my throat, I called her, still unsure it was a wise decision. While I loathed confrontation, did I owe it to our friendship to say something? The easy thing would have been to leave her be, to let the friendship go because I wasn't sure if there was a friendship to salvage. Ultimately, I decided that honesty and solving problems was the best way to go. But she wanted to be absolved; I could feel it. If we talked, it was going to be for *my* benefit, to voice *my* side. So what would I say? *Hey, I got your letter and what a cop-out.*

After the phone rang and Lily answered, I cleared my throat and said, "Maybe we should get together." I didn't want to have our talk over the phone, believing it was best to see each other. She greeted me happily and agreed to go out for coffee.

When Lily came to pick me up from my parents' home, she was surprised at how well I could get around with standing and walking.

Lily aimed for small talk when we sat down on the plush couch at the coffee shop, cups of coffee warming our hands.

It was too much for me. "I can't do this," I said, letting my frustration pour out. "I can't pretend and make small talk."

She sat in silence as I explained my disappointment in her, and how I had barely seen her during such a hard time in my life. What I couldn't say was, *what is wrong with you? How could you send me a letter after years of friendship? I lost my legs. I was burnt to a crisp. I would never do this to you. I'm hurt.*

She tried to explain, as she did in the letter, "There was so much going on in my life then. And there were people who came to visit you and knew exactly what to do. I didn't know what to do." Lily's face was smooth, serene.

Something was missing in this visit. When I saw her at Christmas, she appeared guilty. It was in her face and the way she wrung her hands. She looked at peace now. Lily had a knack for repressing things she found unpleasant. If she was afraid, she pushed fear aside and covered it with a smile. I realized I had fallen into both categories of unpleasant and fear.

"You could have just been there for me. That would have been enough."

And then I retreated, seeing it was futile. She had made up her mind. *This is over.* The letter and her lack of presence in my life made that clear.

I let her off the hook, my turn to cop out. This wasn't worth fighting for, and in that moment of silence, we became mere acquaintances. We caught up on the banal and insignificant, steering ourselves to safety.

While we sat beside each other on either end of the couch, I picked at a sore spot on the inside of my left wrist. There were small white scars going every which way, created by shattered glass from the car. The marks were faint except for one in the center of my wrist directly under the palm of my hand. It was red and irritated. For months this spot had hurt and had grown hard. As Lily and I talked, I rubbed at this spot again, and this time I felt something sharp.

I looked down and saw glass, shiny and clear, poking out of my skin. A year and a half after the crash the last piece of it had worked its way to the surface.

"Oh!" I started to explain, "This is a piece of glass leftover from the car." I waved my wrist at Lily, her face blank.

I picked out the rest of the glass which was the size of a grain of rice. A small reminder of where I'd come from had forced its way out, and I felt its significance as I rolled the jagged glass back and forth, a piece of my past, between my thumb and forefinger.

I wanted to tell someone, someone who'd get it.

When I arrived at my parents' home I showed my mom the piece of glass, like a child with a new toy. "Mom, check this out!"

And then I picked up the phone and called Scott. "You'll never believe it." Before he could respond I filled him in. "Do you know that sore spot under my wrist?"

"Yeah?"

"Well, I was talking to Lily. Remember we were having coffee today? While we were talking, I pulled out a piece of glass."

"No way. What do you think? Windshield? Side window?"

I laughed and sat down hard on the bed. "Crazy, hey? The last piece of the car, the last piece of the accident."

Maybe it was no coincidence to see Lily and have this piece of glass push its way out at the same time. I had given up on 'meant to be,' but I took this as a sign, a whisper in my ear. Today was a day to let go of things that hurt.

I wanted to see Lily, express how I felt and walk on. Our trip to the coffee shop was the last time we went out together. I ran into her from time to time. Civility filled in the distance she created and I continued it, so when we saw each other everything was fine between us.

~~~

The day had come, the day I would officially get another piece of my independence back. I pulled into the Driver Services parking lot and worried I might not pass the test. I felt like I was seventeen again, biting my nails, wondering if I'd screw up.

The man testing me had his eyes on the road and a clipboard in his hands. He only spoke when he directed me, and I kept my hands at ten and two on the steering wheel. I signaled and shoulder-checked my way through his directions. I did not attempt small talk.

We pulled into the parking lot and I shut off the car engine. He wrote on his clipboard as I tried to relax and not squirm in my seat. He looked up. "You've got a few small bad habits left over from years of driving."

I interrupted him, eager to please. "Like what?"

"Like you should signal for longer before changing lanes, but you are good to go."

I ripped the key from the ignition and climbed out of the car. *Is he sure? It can't be that easy.* I followed him into the Driver Services building.

I smiled for the camera and was issued a temporary license until I got a permanent one in the mail. I could drive again. It was redemption. I was free.

I found driving alone in my car therapeutic. I always had. I could put on whatever music I wanted, turn the volume up and drive. My surroundings are a tonic for whatever is bothering me, whether it's the trees reaching toward the sky, the sun finding me through the window and resting on my cheek, or sticking my hand out the window and running my fingers through the air.

Healing didn't come zinging from the sky, zapping me like lightning. It came quietly. I noticed trees against the sky, the lines of the leaves, the sun's glow and how it peeked through the clouds. When twilight came, I remembered why it was my favorite time of the day. Dusk was where day and night joined, meeting up in the sky to curve around each other, bathing the earth in soft pink and orange light. All was right with the world when twilight arrived for me, melodious and serene, a gift.

Joy tiptoed in sweet and gentle, stealing grief from me, until there were mornings I woke up and looked forward to the day ahead of me. It became less about what was not there and more about what remained. Joy was me dancing in the car again, waving my hands in the air, fingers drumming on the steering wheel, singing with gusto, stopping everything at a light so no one could catch me in the act, and then resume dancing when the light turned green.

When the sun and wind found me through the open windows of my car, longing did, too. Some of the old, the 'before' was returning to me. Or that's what I thought it was for a while. But it wasn't the old. It was *me*. I was resurfacing. I saw love, joy, longing, and a piece of glass as markers, showing me how far I'd come, and encouraging me to keep going—that it would be worth it.

24

The Driver

Settlement: an award for being in a car crash.

It was also called compensation, as if there was such a thing. Settlement meant agreement and finality, a summary of everything that happened put to a dollar amount.

I couldn't get used to it. It had been talked about since my parents got a lawyer soon after the crash. I had completed counseling, finished my tests at vocational counseling. Numbers were given to me by my lawyer over the phone and in meetings. One million was as much as the insurance company could offer. There was talk of two, but that was quickly stamped out. There wasn't sufficient coverage in my insurance for that much. My lawyer and the insurance company were coming to an agreement of one million dollars.

I was awarded one million with 20% going to my lawyer. It was a large sum, but when I factored in the cost of legs over my entire life, I was warned it could go fast. I found out that Pharmacare, a government plan that helps British Columbia residents with eligible prescription drugs and designated medical supplies, covers a percentage of these costs. Prosthetics, liners, and repairs add up to thousands of dollars. A pair of legs can cost up to thirty thousand dollars. A portion of that is covered by the government.

My plan was to buy a small house and a car, and to do something for my parents. They had lost wages being with me in the hospital, and had looked after me all my life. They were my parents, and the least I could do was buy them a car. The rest I would save.

I found all of it exhausting, as I did almost everything in the year and a half following the crash. I knew settlement was important, but I don't think I knew how much then. My world was so narrow.

Everything was a step at a time, a day at a time. I didn't think
ahead. I couldn't. It served me well to think and live short term.
To do anything else made me feel as though I would lose grip on
reality, on the here and now. I had always been like this,
thinking weeks and months rather than years. But never was I
more present than I was now.

I knew crashes like mine were the reason we pay for
insurance, but I felt guilty talking money and taking money.
Betty's life could not be bought. To give the crash and its
aftermath value like this seemed wrong. But it was necessary. I
would be hard pressed to find work at that time in my life, or in
the years to come, since I exhausted easily. Going to school
wouldn't be an easy task because I couldn't sit for more than an
hour at a time.

With my settlement, I bought a car for me and a car for my
parents. I would soon begin looking for a house I could call my
own.

While pieces of me were coming back together, I was still
weak and needed a lot of rest. I had my future and my legs to
consider. This injury would always be with me. Other burn
survivors told me that it could take years to have my energy
restored, and even then it may never come back. Few people had
the heart to tell me that I'd never be the same.

My relief this was coming to an end was short-lived.

~~~

"Kevin's coming to see us."

"Do you know what you want to do?" Scott asked.

I got off the phone and eased myself onto my living room
couch. "I'm not sure," I said, drawing a shaky breath. "I know
he'll ask me to go to the trial. I don't know that I can do it...if I
can sit and listen to it all. I just want to live my life and be done
with all of this. I don't know that I want to see the driver. I want
nothing to do with him. Everyone asks if I'm angry at him. I
don't know that I'm angry. I don't want to be angry. I don't
know that he's worth getting angry over. Mostly, I feel nothing."

I was silent for a moment and then said, "If I'm at the trial, it will all come up again, everything I'm working so hard to put behind me."

"I know. Whatever you decide to do, I'm behind you."

Police detective Kevin Wright came with purpose and a thick sheaf of papers under his arm. Jeff, the confirmed driver, was being charged with dangerous driving causing death, and dangerous driving causing bodily harm.

He sat across from me and Scott. "Will you come to the trial?"

"I don't know if I can."

"I know," Kevin said. "I understand this is hard. But we need you there. It's important to put a face to this. You need to be there."

On November 23, 1998 Detective Kevin Wright came on the case, six months after the crash, after the previous investigator returned to his regular duties. I knew Kevin had spent hours on the case working from an anonymous tip to get to the truth, to unravel the lie the brothers told. The detective had photos from ICBC (Insurance Corporation of British Columbia) of his brother showing seatbelt injuries to his neck and chest that were consistent with the marks of a passenger, evidence to bring Kevin a step closer to the truth.

In December, seven months after the crash, Kevin began to call the younger brother, wearing him down until he came to the police station. He told him he had a few questions, assuring him it would only take a few minutes. What was supposed to be a few short minutes turned into an hour with Kevin questioning him until he confessed and announced that his brother Jeff was the driver.

Now that Kevin had the confession, he could focus all his attention on the true driver and build his case. On a cold, icy January morning, the detective waited in his car near Jeff's house. He felt sure that Jeff was still driving, in spite of the fact that he'd been banned from getting behind the wheel. He watched Jeff leave his house, car keys in hand, and climb into his car. He turned the ignition and drove his car down the street toward Kevin, where he stopped Jeff and arrested him.

Jeff was released that same day, on January 22, 1999, eight months after the crash, with a notice to appear in court on March 31, 1999.

As Kevin filled in the blanks, catching me up on all that had happened since the crash, my hesitation wavered. Maybe I shouldn't stay away. Thirty-two witnesses had been interviewed by the police and a 254-page report was sent to Crown Counsel[1] recommending Jeff be charged. I remember telling a reporter that it had been a long year, and I just wanted to leave things alone. I'd meant it then, and everything in me now still wanted to duck for cover under those words. I didn't know how much I could take of this never-ending story. I longed to shut the book, close the door, and turn my back on all of it.

But my feelings changed as I listened to Kevin talk about the police officers who first arrived on scene. They talked about the total chaos and how it looked like a war zone. I heard again how the boys were belligerent and cursing when questioned. We got in *their* way.

Two hours after they slammed into my car, the young men were taken to the hospital by ambulance, accompanied by the police. While talking to them, the officer thought he smelled alcohol on the driver's breath and requested a blood sample. The supposed driver refused and was then charged with refusal, which meant he was given a notice to appear in court. His refusal bought the young men time to hide behind their lie, to tell their friends they would get away

[1] Crown counsels are prosecutors who work for British Columbia's prosecution service—the Criminal Justice Branch of the Ministry of Attorney General. The Criminal Justice Branch operates independently of government and within the justice system. They do not represent the government, the police or the victim of an offence. The courts have described the role of Crown counsel in Canada as a quasi-judicial function and a matter of significant public duty. In our system of justice, when a crime is committed against a victim, it is also a crime against our society as a whole. Therefore, prosecutors do not represent individual victims; they perform their function on behalf of the community.

with it. They stalled, and it almost worked. They didn't count on my parents, the local papers tracking the story, and a dedicated detective, who all worked to get to the truth.

And now here we were, a year later, the driver had finally been charged, and a trial was coming. Although the dates for the trial hadn't been set and could still be a long way off, my commitment was important. Should I do it? Could they count on me?

I knew my parents had fought hard to make this happen, calling the police department for updates, looking for answers, demanding they do their job. While I lay in a hospital bed, broken, justice and heartache were on their minds. I knew Kevin had worked hard to get this case to trial. I wanted to make Kevin Wright's hard work count. I needed to be brave.

"Okay," I said. "I'll come."

25

Betty

A date had not been set for the trial yet, so I pushed it from my mind to make room for other things. A small surgery was coming up, and I was pleased to have a schedule that wasn't filled with moving from one appointment to the next. Life became my own again.

As I returned to the world walking taller, chin higher, the loss of my friend wound its way from the safe recesses of my mind and landed squarely into my heart. Survival and surgery had left little room to mourn her, and I was careful, mindful, of when I let Betty in. If I opened up to her loss all at once, I'd crumple, fall, and not get up. She was always there with me; her presence was never far away. While I fought, her arms were around me. When I made progress, our cheeks pressed against each other in joy.

I ached when my birthday arrived because she would never celebrate another birthday. I wished I could lift her from the photographs on the hospital wall and bring her to life, to hear her voice as she told me about her day. I wouldn't ever watch another movie with her. We wouldn't ever stay up late, our eyelids drooping and fighting sleep to say one more thing.

As I lay on a bed in the holding room, waiting for someone to take me into surgery, the loss of Betty grew from an ache to anguish. The procedure I was having was to reduce the scar beside my chin. This was the last surgery of all the surgeries, and I would be in and out within hours.

The curtain that separated me from the rest of the room pulled to the side, the rings scraping along the metal rod. "All right, let's go." A nurse looked at me expectantly.

"Umm..." I started to sit up, to explain.

"Well? Are you getting into the bed?" She looked bored and moved the gurney closer. I guessed she thought if the words weren't helping maybe the visual of the gurney would convey the urgency of getting into the bed.

"Um, I can't. I'm...I'm an amputee and I don't have my legs on." I still had trouble saying the word *amputee*. I had to force it out, and the words threatened to stick in my throat. "My prosthetic legs have been put away because of the surgery, and I can't get to them."

"Oh! I'm so sorry!" She continued to apologize as she moved the gurney right next to my bed, so I could scoot on over.

I smiled. "It's okay."

She talked to me as she wheeled me to surgery. "Honey, how did this happen?"

Maybe it was our shared embarrassment, or her having moved from apologizing to sincerity when she asked; or maybe it was that I was naked, stripped of my legs with only a thin gown to protect me that allowed me to let my guard down. My eyes were free of contact lenses and created a warped, blurred view of my nurse, which made me feel especially vulnerable. Seconds passed, and I found myself crying, overcome as I told her about the car crash. *But the worst part, the worst part was that my best friend died.*

Grief sprung up when I least expected it. Just when I thought I had a handle on it, just when I thought I was doing so well, it surged through me and leaked from my nose, my eyes, and rolled down my cheeks and into my hair.

I didn't attend Betty's funeral. I couldn't. I was unconscious, in surgery, unaware as people came together to mourn the loss of Betty's light on earth. The funeral was held in a large church, large enough to hold the many people who knew her, loved her, and wanted to be close to her one last time. Songs were sung, prayers given, and benedictions offered as people remembered and cried, stricken by the speed and ferocity of her death.

Metal against metal, Betty was pushed into death. It came quickly. We weren't ready.

Was there a signal missed, a warning felt in the pit of the stomach, a prickling at the back of the neck that this was coming? Something to whisper that loss is near. Loss you cannot prepare for. Would that change anything? If I had known, would we have argued a week before the crash? Would I have reminded you that I loved you? Would I have done everything in my power to cushion the blow? We say that if we knew, we would have, could have, should have.

Betty knew I loved her. We had an argument about my seeing her less when I started seeing Scott. I wasn't around as much. She was hurt, and I was defensive. We were conflicted, but it didn't change our friendship. I didn't stop saying she was like the sister I never had.

We were on our way to a restaurant to say our goodbyes. Betty was leaving town for the summer and would be working as a camp counselor. We never made it to the restaurant. We didn't know we would be saying goodbye in a church, in a hospital, and every day in the months to follow.

As the youngest in the family, Betty had the protective eyes of her four older brothers and her father watching over her. She was only fourteen when she and her mother were in a car crash that tragically killed her mother.

I was sixteen and went to her mom's funeral, and watched her family walk down the aisle, hunched over with grief.

Betty and I became friends after high school, through boy breakups. We were both getting over a guy. We always said if it wasn't for those guys we may have never become friends. We shared clothes and opinions. We talked fast and used our hands for emphasis. We spent hours poring over our lives, what we would be, who we could become. Our destinies were still unwritten, and we were excited by our prospects.

Betty was an incredible listener. She was so engaged, her eyes trained on you, and nothing diverted her attention. She had a ready, loud laugh that turned into a guffaw when she was genuinely amused or delighted. She was compassionate, and effortless in it. When I lived on my own and was in between jobs, low on cash and food, she showed up at my doorstep with bags of groceries in her hands. "For you!" she said happily. "And I don't want to hear a word about it."

I could rarely say no to the gleam in her eye, to her ideas that promised adventure. She forced me to watch *Beaches;* a movie I thought would be too sappy for me. As the credits rolled I sat up on the couch, wiping the tears from my eyes, and sighed. "All right, I loved it. You got me."

One evening she begged me to go somewhere, anywhere with her. "Let's just drive and see where the road takes us!" We drove until a storm forced us to take shelter in a run-down motel for the night. The fun wasn't ruined, not when we had access to greasy cheesy fries, colts (small flavored cigars), and reruns of the original *Beverly Hills 90210*. Betty always brimmed with possibility and saw potential everywhere.

She never let me say a bad word against my mother. Not when her own mother had been ripped from her. I would be irritated with my mom, grumbling at something she said that rubbed me the wrong way, and Betty would chastise me, saying, "You have a mom," stressing the mom. "You should be thankful." She said this with wide eyes and a calm don't-mess-with-me kind of way.

Betty reminded me of the good in my life. I think that's why she chastised—to remind me of what could happen, what I could lose so easily. She knew. And she would do what she could to protect me.

Two weeks before the crash, we met at a park one evening and went for a walk. She had just returned from the cemetery. "I went to see my mom this afternoon."

"How was that?" I asked. I looked at her; I knew this face, a face open and easy to read.

Her lips pressed in a thin line, she was pensive, thoughtful. "It was good. Really good. It felt different visiting her this time. More..." She seemed to search for the right words. "It was peaceful.

I felt at peace. Like I could finally let her go…like it was okay to let her go." She linked her arm through mine.

"Oh Betty, that's so…" I couldn't find the right word, a word to describe something so sacred. A word to encompass all she had gone through. To let go of her mom was something I didn't dare speak to because I wasn't able to understand a loss that deep. I squeezed her arm and whispered, "I'm happy for you. I love you."

"I'm happy for me, too." We walked arm in arm until we reached the playground and made our way to the swings. We sat side by side, our legs and arms dangling, enjoying the sunset, and the gentle creak of the swings.

In the blink of an eye, the trigger had been pulled, and we were blindsided by that car. The car hit the passenger side, her side. She, with no choice, was my shield. Her body protected my own as my car spun across the intersection, plowed through a fence, tumbled down a ravine, and landed upside down at the bottom. If it wasn't for the car catching fire, I would have come away with scratches, a few broken ribs, and a collapsed lung.

Betty, age twenty-one, destiny unfulfilled, died on impact.

I tried to make sense of a life cut short. I demanded answers and attempted to make the pieces fit. But they didn't. They couldn't. Life ended swiftly, and there was no rationale to it. Why did people say there must be a reason? There was no reason, and I was tired of hearing how there must be some cosmic logic to her death, that maybe we wouldn't know the reason here on earth, but one day it would be made known to us in Heaven. I didn't understand what that meant. Life was *here, now,* and why wait for Heaven to give me some wisdom?

So, I reasoned. I tried. I made. I learned.

I grieved and celebrated.

I wanted order, and found it in the chaos. I was guilty of being alive. I didn't have the answers for *why me* and *why her?* Why didn't she get to live? I could not answer that question, and never would. Life did what it wanted, favoring the unpredictable. I would have to choose how I was going to live. I followed my instinct to persevere, and did what I could to survive tragic losses and a life cut short. I could choose hope over bitterness, or bitterness over hope. I could accept. And that was the hardest part. *The surrendering.* To stretch out my hands, palms up, and take in the loss. Death came unbidden, and I had to accept and accept and accept until it was a part of me, woven and stitched to me.

I thought about the day I heard Betty's funeral on a cassette tape. Her brother brought it to the hospital and sat with me while I listened. Angela was there, too. I heard the songs and the words.

I looked at her brother as if through warped glass. How could this happen? To him? To his family? Again. Losing his mom, and then his sister like this. He shouldn't have to do this, to be here, but he was here, and I was humbled. Everything was wavy and blurred, the colors washed out. My grief was far away, untouchable. Betty's death wasn't final for me. Still so caught up in her life, it went on and on, whether she was here or not.

I saw Betty everywhere. She was in my closet, her sweater folded on the shelf, her dress on a hanger, skimming the floor. She was in the long limbs of a young woman at the mall, in the tilt of a woman's head in conversation with a friend, and in the dark wavy hair of another. My heart raced and hope rose as I craned my neck for a closer look, only to shake my head, remembering that she isn't here and would never be here. I kept walking, wondering if anyone else saw my flushed face and the way my hands shook. Sometimes I felt her laugh, her presence, around me. I didn't care if it was real, or if I made it up. It comforted me to think of her as being around. Her joy had always been so contagious. Why couldn't it still be here affecting me, nudging me in the right direction?

Betty and I grew up on God, Church, and Faith. Eternity was a promise. Betty believed in Heaven. It was where her mother came to rest. Eternity was a beautiful word, a peaceful place, and I hoped it was real. I pictured Betty reunited with her mother, safe and contented.

Betty's short life demanded celebrating, and I wanted to honor her by loving her, by remembering her. She was still here because her soul was imprinted on the people who loved her. I knew the brush of death, its icy fingers, its sour smell, and alarming stillness, but after traveling through the cold passage of death, I knew she was greeted with light. Betty belonged in Eternity, in a life everlasting. There were still tears in my eyes as the nurse held my hand.

The doctor's voice was soft. "Breathe deeply, Heidi."

I drew a deep breath. Betty. My sweet friend.

"Count down from 10."

I miss you.

"10, 9, 8, 7, 6..."

The light and floating feeling came. My head felt disconnected from the rest of me, bobbing like a balloon.

"Breathe deeply. Thatta girl."

By the time I reached 3, I was on my way to the dark to rest.

26
I Do

Scott and I sat on a park bench at Vanier Park discussing the validity of soul mates. Was there such a thing?

"I don't know if I believe in soul mates," I said. "How is it that your soul mate always ends up living near or in the same town as you?"

"Yeah, I don't know that I believe in soul mates, either," letting the word roll off his tongue like it was a joke. "One person. Forever."

I laughed. "It's perfect until someone dies and then you have to find a new soul mate."

Nearby, a kite ducked and soared. I shielded my face from the wind and turned to him. "I think it's a choice."

"When this first happened, your parents told me I could leave, that they would understand if I left. I could see the fork in the road, you know? I could have left. I knew it would be easier to walk away, but I'd always be wondering 'what if.' So, I chose the path with you. I wanted to see how you'd do."

I nodded knowingly. "I don't know if we're destined to be, but with all that's happened, it does sometimes feel like we're meant to be together. I mean, we got serious so fast and then this happened…" I tossed my hands in the air.

I watched boats bob up and down in the ocean and thought about my future, our future. "There's no one I'd rather do this with."

We sat shoulder to shoulder, our hands and fingers entwined, easy in our shared doubt toward soul mates and the knowledge that if there was such a thing, this was the closest we'd be to it.

It was Valentine's Day, a year and a half after the crash, when Scott got down on one knee and proposed to me at the fountain outside of Queen Elizabeth Theater. It was a cold night and bundled-up strangers walked by and clapped as they witnessed the proposal and my squealed, "Yes!" He slipped the ring onto my finger, a ring that matched the promise ring he gave me on my birthday.

After we were engaged I began to barrage him with questions. I wanted to know what he would be like when we got married. I had heard stories of men changing as soon as they walked down the aisle, and I swore that would not happen to me. I gave him scenarios and asked what his responses would be in different situations. Scott sighed and answered the questions.

"This is what you do."

"What do I do?"

"There's a big change, and you get scared."

"I'm not scared." I backtracked. "Okay, I'm a little scared. What if we don't like living together?"

Our plan was to move in together after we got married. With part of the settlement, I had bought a townhouse in Langley, about forty-five minutes east of Vancouver. He lived in a basement suite with a friend.

"We'll be fine. We'll learn as we go. And with me, what you see is what you get. There are no surprises."

I searched his face. When I was at G.F. Strong I made sure I wanted to be with him. Even though we were surviving something terrible together, I didn't want to be with him because no one else wanted me. I had to be able to stand on my own, that I was good enough without a man. As great as it was that Scott stuck with me, I needed to be sure I wanted to be stuck with him.

We were engaged, another step towards forever. And that wasn't said dreamily, with visions of a bride and groom perched at the top of a six-tiered wedding cake. It was with reality, with startling clarity, that I realized we were going to be making vows to each other, promising to be together against all the odds. I wanted us to be sure this was it.

War had bound us together and cemented our love. We got to know each other in the darkest places and came through to the other side. From the moment I met Scott, I knew peace. He was serene and steadfast, my sanctuary. If we could survive hell, we could weather the trials of marriage. I wanted to walk through this world with him. If there was such a thing as soul mate, Scott was it. He understood me, he got me, and that was enough for me to say yes.

~~~

Married friends warned me I might not remember the day, it goes so fast. Try to be present. Enjoy the day, they said. While I might not remember every detail, I knew this would be an incredible day. Even if I couldn't recall the color of the flowers, I knew I would remember Scott waiting for me at the end of the aisle and how sure I felt as I said, "I do."

On November 4, 2000 I slipped on my white Keds, lacing them up with light pink ribbon to make my feet pretty. The shoes needed to be flat and light. Heels were not an option.

As I put on my dress and my friends and bridesmaids, Loraleigh and Angela, tied the corset at my back, I was transformed. I was in love with my dress of ivory and the lightest shade of pink, and embroidered with flowers. Except for the excited whirling in my stomach, I didn't feel sick. Better yet, I didn't look sick, even though I wore pressure garments over my patchwork quilt of scars. But this day, I would not be consumed by that. Today I was a young woman getting married.

It was a new day, a celebration of love, life, and commitment. I had been lost, and today I felt found. Scott and I were changed and battle-weary, but we were also strong and secure in our love and hope. Hope for a long future because of a past we endured together.

On our way to the church, I thought about Betty and how she should be with us, dressing up, laughing, and rushing out the door as one of my bridesmaids. I was comforted that we lit a candle in her honor at the front of the church. I wanted her there with me.

Clutching my bouquet, I took a short second to soak up my elation to be walking down the aisle. No wheelchair, no canes; I vibrated with happiness. I felt beautiful.

I stood at the doors, my hand on my dad's arm and waited for my cue.

"All rise."

This is it. I held on to my dad as I walked down the aisle to face Scott, to speak our vows in front of nearly two hundred guests.

It was a short ceremony. I loathed going to long and drawn out weddings where the officiate usurped the ceremony and made it less about the bride and groom and more about the message he wanted to deliver. I had the same philosophy for the reception, and didn't want too many speeches. Scott's parents spoke, and Jodi, Scott's sister, read a lovely poem she had written. My parents stood at the microphone together as my dad spoke in a warm voice.

He recalled me as a baby, how I often had my fists up, already a fighter. "That became Heidi's trademark, and she never gave up easily." He finished by saying, "We're very proud of both you and Scott."

I squeezed Scott's hand under the table. "We're married."

He smiled his crooked smile, the one I thought was so cute when we went out for the first time. "I'm happy. Are you?"

"Very."

When the food was served and everyone was busy eating, Scott's cousins handed Scott his childhood Superman cape. "I didn't know this still existed!" he laughed while draping it across his shoulders.

"It suits you," I laughed, imagining his four-year-old self pretending to fly through the house, leaping tall buildings in a single bound. With or without the cape, I realized he was a superhero, and had been for the last two years.

The reception was nearly over, and I wanted to talk to Loraleigh and Angela one last time before we left. "Did you feel her here?" I didn't have to explain 'her.' They knew.

"I think she was here with us," Angela said.

Loraleigh agreed. "Could you feel her, Heidi?"

I nodded. We smiled at each other, our eyes shining with tears. Understanding borne over years of friendship, we didn't need words to share how we could almost hear Betty's laughter, see her eyes widen as she leaned close to tell a story, and express how much we missed her. I hugged them goodbye. "I love you guys."

It was time to go. I turned to find Scott, to take his hand and walk to the car, guests calling out goodbyes and congratulations under the evening sky. I laughed as Scott tied his cape and threw it over his shoulder with a flourish. I batted my eyes in mock worship. "My hero."

He was my hero, not because he was perfect, but because he stood with me. Even in fear, he never ran. He promised me love would get me through, even when I was unsure that love would be enough. Looking in his eyes, seeing his small smile, I knew love would be enough. Here on this day, surrounded by family and friends, I was loved. I didn't know what else life would throw at us, but whatever came, I could trust love. I could trust him.

In just a few days, we would be on our way to Ireland, then Scotland, on our way to another beginning. Life, we discovered, was full of them.

27
The Trial

Four years after the crash, Jeff's trial began. For four years, Jeff had been free. Scott and I had been married for nearly two years when the impending trial became a cloud over my life. While I had perfected crossing bridges when I was thrown onto them, the cloud loomed larger and larger in my life until it was all I could see.

The trial was set to last a week and Jeff, the driver, chose to have a trial by judge rather than by jury. I couldn't testify because I had no recollection of the day. Instead, my body told the story I couldn't.

I walked into the courthouse looking for the board that would direct me to the room we'd be in for the day. I skimmed over the lists on the wall, searching for his last name. To see his name in print, to know we were about to embark on his fate left me hollow. Our lives were intertwined. If he wasn't found guilty, did that mean I was guilty? The entire day was wiped from my memory and left at the bottom of a ravine. Did I see them coming? For half a second did I look left instead of right when I crossed the street? I still doubted that I should be here, and worried the anatomy of the crash would open wounds I had just sewn up. I was a robot that morning, numb and detached, going through the motions of doing what I was told and fulfilling my promise to the detective.

I found the room and made my way toward the back, seeking distance from the driver. The room was smaller than I thought it would be, so it was impossible to hide. But I knew how to retreat, to hide within, to survive. As I sat and waited, sitting on my ice-cold hands to stop them from shaking, I wondered what Jeff looked like. I had never even seen a photo of him, never asked questions about him, so I didn't know what to expect.

The small room filled with people. With my dad sitting beside me, we waited soundlessly. The small hard knot in my stomach grew bigger with every minute that passed, and I was nauseous with fear of the unknown. Would he be proven guilty? I wished we were at the end. I wished I could hear the verdict. I wished I didn't have to be in the same room with him. A young man sat down at the front of the room, his back toward us. I whispered to my dad, "Is that him?" He nodded and cleared his throat.

Jeff sat up straight. His light hair cut short, he was clean-shaven, and wore a button down shirt with a collar. I expected something different, someone sinister, someone who looked like a bad guy. I was struck by his ordinariness.

The murmuring in the room stopped as the judge took his seat. Predictably, Jeff's plea was not guilty.

Crown Counsel called the first witness. No backing out now. I'm in for the long haul.

Witness after witness came up to speak about what they had seen or hadn't seen, until their testimonies blurred together. *Yes, I saw him speeding. No, I can't say that I remember. We were racing and then we slowed down, we pulled back. It's a busy road. Well, I don't know that it's that busy. It depends on the day. I saw his car fishtail.*

The day's proceedings ended swiftly and were irresolute. I couldn't keep track of what had transpired. If I felt the testimonies were wish-washy, would the judge feel that way, too? Everything I fought to keep out suddenly poured in. Jeff and his brother's arrogance and their lies against Betty and me cut holes in my armor and crawled under my skin. I wanted to plead with these witnesses. Don't you know what he's done? *I look fine now, but I wasn't fine four years ago. I nearly died, and my best friend is buried. Because of him.*

I understood the witnesses' reluctance and uncertainty. So much time had passed. Memory lost its color, details slipped, and it was scary to know that each word you speak could be held against someone else. But Jeff wasn't on trial for an *accident*. He wouldn't be here if this was an accident. He was here because he broke laws and lied to escape those laws. I knew he didn't get up that morning intending to kill someone, but we were victims of his choice. The brothers were calloused as they cursed at us while our bodies were on fire. I knew I would feel differently, more compassionate, if he had shown remorse, if he hadn't lied. I just didn't understand his reactions, or how a person could do this to another person. Fury coursed through me. My legs prickled with pain, my skin screamed, and my heart raced as every truth made my heart beat faster.

Crown Counsel stuck to the facts so some of the details I had come to know weren't spoken out loud. They did this to keep emotion out, only allowing the facts to prove his guilt. I was spent when I went home that day, hit hard with emotion and afraid the facts wouldn't be enough.

The next day, after police reports and more facts, I was in the courthouse bathroom washing my hands at the sink when I noticed a familiar face beside me that I quickly recognized as Jeff's girlfriend.

I'd heard he had a girlfriend. She sat near the front, close to him. I wondered what compelled someone to stay with a person like him. What kind of woman was she that she could support his actions?

I averted my eyes in case she knew me. A part of me wanted to say something, to acknowledge the awfulness of our situation, of both our positions. But what could I say to her that wouldn't be awkward, that could sum up years' worth of a fight I wished I'd never had to wage? This wasn't her fight. She was there to support him, and there was nothing to say. I didn't know if she recognized me. I hurriedly rinsed my hands to escape the small room and the nearness of her. Of him.

I returned to our room for the day and sat down next to my mom. I spoke quietly, under my breath. "I was just in the bathroom with Jeff's girlfriend. I'm surprised she's with him, that anyone would be with him. Maybe he's changed?"

Maybe he had admitted his guilt and taken responsibility, allowing time to temper him. And then I remembered his not guilty plea. I didn't give my mom a chance to speak. "You know what? I don't think I can talk about this." Already he took up more room, more air than he should, and it was getting harder to keep him out. This was exactly what I wanted to avoid, why I didn't want to go to the trial. He was everywhere and he had a life. He moved on when my friend couldn't. He got a job and a girlfriend while I painfully pieced my life back together. The distance I worked hard to maintain between us was threatened.

I shut my eyes to shut him out.

I saw rather than felt anger, crimson and pulsing. I dug my nails into my palms to distract my racing mind and get through the rest of the day. She nodded and patted my knee. It was almost time to go home, and we were already anticipating the next day's rounds. It was the engineer's turn to testify, and we knew this would be the testimony that would count.

The next day, the judge leaned in as we listened to the engineer's testimony confirm that I could have never seen Jeff coming. All the angst I'd carried through the week disappeared, my body relaxed for the first time in days as I listened to his report.

Skid marks proved that the laws of physics were against me. The engineer assessed that Jeff's vehicle was traveling at a minimum speed of 106 to 115 km/h at the initiation of skidding activity. This would be *after* he applied the brakes, which meant his speed before hitting the brakes was even higher. The estimated speed at impact was 92 to 101km/h.

The engineer's estimates were conservative to leave no room for doubt. The maximum speed he was traveling could have been as high as 150km/h. That equals 95 miles per hour.

At that speed, it was impossible for me to have seen him coming when I left the stop sign. I couldn't have slowed down or sped up, and was an inevitable target. If he had stepped on the brakes earlier, even going over the 60 km/h speed limit by 10 to 20 km/h, we would have missed one another. There was nothing I could have done.

As the engineer spoke, I felt lighter, liberated. I wanted to cry. After years of bad news, a life disrupted and a life gone, we had good news. After a long hunt for the truth, it was claimed, here with us. I had no hand in my friend's death.

Later that night, my newfound freedom vanished, and I couldn't sleep. I was riddled with doubt. I heard the report, but what if the judge saw it differently? What if there wasn't enough evidence? I had no memory of that day, so what if I'm guilty? Even by just a small percent?

The verdict would be announced tomorrow. Scott and I had already speculated about the day, deciding our lives would go on regardless of the verdict. We had the truth now. But that verdict mattered to me. I had gone to the trial because Kevin Wright asked me to go, but as the week unfolded, my need for justice grew. I didn't want Jeff to be let off the hook, to escape the consequences and be rewarded for his lie. While Scott slept beside me, I was consumed with the verdict that would be handed down in that courtroom, and how our lives would be impacted yet again. It was hours before I finally drifted into a fitful sleep.

I arrived in court the next morning and went to my usual spot at the back. A family friend greeted my mom and me with daffodils, bouquets of hope. I lay the flowers across my lap and watched the door, waiting for the judge to appear.

Within seconds a hush fell over the room. As he entered, I sucked in my breath and chewed on the insides of my cheeks, searching his face for clues. *Guilty, not guilty?* His face remained smooth and passive as he sat down. *Please, just blurt it out. Guilty, not guilty.*

As the judge spoke I held my breath, hands curled into fists, my nails digging into my palms. I didn't hear anything until, "Guilty."

I let out my breath in a whoosh and released my nails from my palms. I didn't want to hug or revel in victory. I shuddered as relief ran through my body.

We got the bad guy.

The prosecutor for Crown Counsel ushered some members of Betty's family, my mom, and I to a small room downstairs afterward, and debriefed. Brian, the prosecutor for Crown Counsel, filled us in on what was coming up next. Sentencing for Jeff would come at a later date, and he wanted to know if we had any requests. Some of Betty's family wanted a facilitated meeting with Jeff.

Brian asked me, "Is this something you want?"

Slow to respond, I shook my head. "I don't think so. I don't have anything to say to him."

Betty's family was more forgiving. I wanted to wash my hands of all of it. I couldn't imagine sitting in a room with him, talking about something neither of us could change. It had taken all I had to go to this trial. I let my guard down and let him in, going against my rule of not giving him more power than he already had. I was already busy rebuilding my armor, constructing the walls to keep me secure. How much of my life could one person claim?

~~~

Sentencing for Jeff came three months after the trial. It certainly wasn't like the movies where everything was hurried along. With one bang of the gavel, it was over.

Victims and family members of the victims were supposed to have Victim Impact Statements prepared for sentencing. The cloud returned dark and foreboding. I had to face him again, and this time the crash would not be reduced to numbers and facts. This day would be dedicated to emotion, to grief. I had confronted anger during the trial, and I knew sentencing would go deeper. This time it would hurt.

I was advised to hold nothing back in my statement, to be completely honest about what I wanted to say to Jeff, to the

court. Perhaps I should arrive in a wheelchair to drive home
what he had done to me. I refused. "I'm walking. I worked too
hard for this only to go back to a chair. He's not taking that away
from me."

I gave myself over to the crash. It was the first time I had written
about it.

I struggled to write about how Jeff's negligence impacted my
life. I would speak these words out loud, and they'd land with a
blow, with finality. I didn't have hours to speak, and I didn't want to
pour out my heart. Although it was the court-appointed time to lay
my soul bare and be vulnerable, I couldn't. I had worked hard to rise
up, to be a survivor, and it was too painful to revert to the role of
victim. As I thought about what I wanted to say and how I couldn't
sum up suffering on one page, my statement turned into more of a
list of all that had gone wrong. It also became about choices—his
choice and how that influenced every choice I made after that for the
rest of my life. Because he wanted to drive fast that day, drive at all
that day, I had to live with his choices. I knew he had to live and
endure the consequences of his choices, too. I knew this wasn't what
he planned. He hadn't planned to harm or kill anyone, but it's what
happened, and it could have been prevented.

And what about after the crash? He had lied. He blamed his
brother. Witnesses overheard them wishing us dead in a fit of fury
over their banged up car. We were "bitches" who had gotten in their
way. People make mistakes, and most of us learn from them. We say
we're sorry and beg for forgiveness. He never apologized. He crowed
around town that he would get away with it. He pled not guilty. I
couldn't push this from my mind as I wrote. A police officer at the
scene said that in all of her career, she had never met suspects as
horrible and callous as Jeff and his brother. She couldn't understand
their behavior, their belligerence, or the way they blamed us.

It wouldn't help to rail against him and allow my anger to cloud
my statement. I needed to be clear and straightforward for the judge,
for me. I pressed my pen to paper and hovered between writing
about how this guy is a colossal jackass, and sticking to the facts.

Clarity won. I could vent my anger through my list of injuries, in my many months spent at the hospital. *This* is what happened. Despite what he's done, I'm still here.

Sentencing was gut-wrenching, worse than the trial. It would be over in hours, but I knew by now that time meant nothing when it came to tearing lives apart.

The room was silent as I walked to the small podium to stand in front of the judge, my back turned to everyone else. I felt calm.

On August 23, 2002, I read:

"I don't remember the accident or the day that it happened. I just know that one day I woke up and everything had changed.

"I came to after being in a drug-induced coma for almost a month. My ribs were broken, puncturing one of my lungs. I had third and fourth degree burns to 52% of my body—fourth degree being to muscle and bone. Because of the severity of the burns, I had a temporary colostomy and my right leg was amputated below the knee. I had many skin grafts, which involved taking skin from my head, my arms, and my back, and grafting it to the rest of my body. There were infections that delayed my healing. Somewhere in all of that, I was told they would also have to amputate my left leg. Each morning I had dressing changes that were excruciating. My showers were so unbearable, they had to anesthetize me.

"I had a body I didn't recognize. I didn't know who I was anymore. I had lost Betty—one of my dearest and closest friends. I was devastated in every way.

"I spent seven months at Vancouver General Hospital in the burn unit, and then five months at a rehabilitation center. In just over a year I had over twenty surgeries.

"Everything is different now—from getting in and out of bed, to grocery shopping, to my perspective on life. As an amputee I use 40-50% more energy than the average person. My legs suffer from serious skin breakdown, which prevents me from being as active as I would like to be. I'll never have a steady job. My prosthetics will always be a financial burden.

"I miss long walks, running, hiking, going to the beach on a hot day. I miss my legs and the freedom and independence they bring. I miss my skin—the body I once had. I will never have that back. This was not something I chose. These were not circumstances I created.

"The results and consequences of June 12, 1998 will continue. I've spent four years surviving and fighting this. So much went from possible to impossible that day. My world came apart in less than a second, and I've returned to an entirely different world."

Electricity surged through me as I read my statement. My face flushed hot and cold. My voice didn't waver. Calm was replaced with passion. Damn this guy. He wasn't even supposed to be driving that day. If he hadn't hit us, it would only be a matter of time before it was someone else he sent to the hospital, someone else killed. Betty is not here, and he didn't care. I was so tired of reining it in, keeping myself in check...for what? For so long I had looked at the crash as this horrible thing that happened. Bad things happen. But I knew I could turn around and point my finger at the cause.

Anger ignited, and I drew power from it. Strength rose in my voice, in my body, as I stood straight, my neck angled toward the single sheet of paper. This wasn't my time to be vulnerable. It was time for me to get angry. I was vast, a giant, as my voice filled the room. I didn't see or hear anyone as I read.

This was not something I chose. These were not circumstances I created.

I finished and watched my feet as I returned to my chair. I would not cry this day. I had shed enough tears over what he had done to me and Betty.

The prosecutor, Brian, read a letter from my parents. My parents were there, but chose to have Counsel read the letter. Betty's sister-in-law represented the entire family, and cried while she spoke of Betty's life, how she was missed, how Betty wouldn't see her young nieces grow, and how her death tainted their view of the future by shattering their world as they knew it. She spoke of forgiveness, of grace, and love.

It was Jeff's turn to speak.

He stood at the front of the room, beside his lawyer, and turned to look at us. It was the first time he had faced us. "I'm sorry. I hope you can forgive me."

My body rigid and my mind numb, I couldn't bring myself to make eye contact with him. I wouldn't forgive him. I looked at my hands. *Who are you doing this for, Jeff? For the judge? For you? Because it couldn't have been for us.* He had years to make this right, to apologize.

We were all in one room—on opposite sides of a large room that smelled of furniture polish and stale perfume. Jeff's family and friends were on the left side of the room and we were on the right. We weren't a big group—Betty's sister-in-law, my parents, Scott and I, Angela, and my friend, Tanya. Most of Betty's family kept their distance, preferring to keep their grief private. I suspected both women in their lives being claimed by car crashes was too painful, too much for them to bear. It was unfathomable to me how this could happen; I couldn't imagine what they had to endure. Twice. When they saw me, I wondered if all they could see was Betty.

After Jeff spoke, the judge excused himself as he deliberated over his decision. We were free to have lunch and wait.

Seated at a café nearby, I picked at my food and chatted with everyone, but I couldn't think beyond what I had written, what waited for us.

As we walked back to the courthouse I glanced up at the sky and took note of the warm clear day, a day for enjoying the sun, a day for fresh air and fun. Not a day like today, a day I wished I would be able to forget.

An hour later the air was sucked out of the room as the judge read his ruling. Jeff stood as the judge sentenced him to one year in prison, prohibited him from driving for five years, and granted mediation at Betty's family's request.

One year.

We had been warned the sentence could have been a stern reprimand of community service. One year in prison wasn't enough, but nothing would have been enough. My head exploded in pain and a bitter taste invaded my mouth. I was dizzy with exhaustion, dizzy with grief, dizzy with all that had led to this day. I had to get out of there. Now.

Jeff was handcuffed and led out of court to the strains of his girlfriend crying out, "I love you!"

We didn't say a word. There was nothing to say. Nobody won. Betty was gone. Jeff was going to prison.

As we filed out of the court room Jeff's brother shouted after us, "You fucking ruined his life!"

I felt like I was stabbed in the back, blood drawn by his accusation. I shook with anger at his words. I didn't look back as Scott and I walked out of the building and to the car. Instead, I kept my eyes trained on every step forward.

Our mood was somber on the way home. I said to Scott, "Could you feel their anger? Not just Jeff's brother, but the whole family? It was palpable. How can they be so angry? We didn't do this. We're all here because of him. We didn't ruin his life. Jeff did."

Scott seemed to have a clearer mind on their reaction. "You didn't go away. Your parents, Betty's family, you. You fought. I don't think they were expecting that."

"That was awful. I didn't know it would feel like that. I thought it would feel like justice was served, that we would feel better, somehow. Vindicated. But it's not like that. It's not like that at all."

"Nothing about this feels good." He said, shaking his head.

The snap of the handcuffs and the *I love you* that rang out in the room clamped down on my heart and haunted me for months. From her side, she was robbed. But in spite of the fact that we were also robbed, my compassion for her pulled me to the middle, and I was confused about how I should feel and where I should stand. So many were wounded. She was hurt. I was hurt. I understood hurt, and I knew I'd never forget that *I love you*.

~~~

The phone rang and I was confused by the caller ID, but I pushed the button to talk. "Hello?"

"Hello. Is this Heidi Kroeker?"

"Yes. Well, I was a Kroeker. Now I'm a Cave."

"Hi, Heidi. This is Victim Services calling. How are you?"

"I'm fine."

"We're calling to let you know that Jeff will be released early on parole."

"Okay." I clutched the phone against my ear. My head began to ache. I quickly counted out the months since he had been in jail. Five months. Barely five months.

"It's mandatory that we call you." The voice was kind. "Do you have any questions?"

"No." Should I? "So, he's just out now?"

"Soon. He'll be released in the next few days."

"Well, thank you for letting me know."

I put the phone down and stared at the calendar I had been marking with plans and things to do. I placed my hand on my still-flat tummy. It was a new reflex after learning I was pregnant in November, already looking after my baby. It was a few days before Christmas.

Should I call someone with the news? Had they contacted Betty's family? I picked up the phone to call Scott and stared at the buttons. Maybe I should call my mom. She'll be upset. She'll say it's too soon. *How can he be out this soon?* I put the phone down.

I felt fragile, which was weird because I rarely felt fragile. I knew what it was to be vulnerable, but I never felt breakable. For a few seconds, I felt like molten glass, afraid to move for fear of changing shape. I needed to be alone with it. Quiet. I reminded myself to breathe.

On the surface, everything looked great, but if someone peered closely, got right in my face, they would see it in my eyes — the hairline fracture. When you're hit hard again and again, a mark is made, one that will stay. He would be out to share Christmas with his loved ones, and I would have to pat that down, make it smooth, because it's out of my hands, and I was desperate to be okay. What can I do? He is out. But for now, for a few minutes, I was pulled apart by the life behind me and the life in front of me, and splintered by sadness.

28

Redemption

When I was in the hospital battling my injuries, the possibility of my having a baby was questioned. The skin across my ribs and down my sides was grafted, and cinched me. The nurses and I were concerned there wasn't enough elasticity in my skin to stretch during pregnancy. There was scarring around my vagina, too, which meant there was a slim-to-zero chance that I could deliver my babies in the conventional way. In fact, there was worry that having sex might be iffy due to possible internal damage where fire and smoke claimed more than my skin.

It was my nurse, Kathleen, whose eyes lit with mischief, sweetly said, "There are other things you can do besides intercourse. If you'd like we could have a counselor speak with you."

Ummm, no way in hell. I knew how to make out with a guy. I didn't need a counselor giving me tips on kissing or being felt up. It was taking sex off the table completely that freaked me out. No sex. Ever? Panicked wasn't adequate for how I felt. I was still a virgin, and it seemed more than cruel that this could be my next twist of fate in this ongoing saga. It was just mean. There was nothing like the loss of limbs, skin, and possibly a vagina to make a guy want to say, oh yeah, you're the girl for me.

I was promised that the next time I was in surgery, a doctor would check me out. I woke up to reassuring words. "It looks like you're going to be fine."

What relief. Sex was back on the table, so to speak. I hung a lot of hope on *fine*, my new favorite word.

I was comforted by Kathleen, who had offered up winks and nudges weeks earlier, when she told me there was enough good skin in the center of my belly to handle the stretch and pull of a growing baby.

I worried I wouldn't become pregnant, not because of scarring, but because life was fickle. I stood in the long shadow of the crash and I wondered if my list of terrible wasn't quite done, that maybe I wouldn't get pregnant because, well, that's life. Things had been pretty even and good for a couple of years now. Maybe it was time for something bad to happen, to balance the good. I knew this way of thinking was a bad trail to follow, and would do little but paralyze me with fear. I was afraid of more suffering, and I didn't want to know the burden of infertility, too.

After trying for six months I became pregnant with my daughter. Fear was pushed back until I began cramping and spotting in my twelfth week. Scared that shadow was growing darker, I went to the hospital. After waiting for hours in emergency, I was reassured when I heard the miracle of her heartbeat, quick and strong. It sounded like the wings of a butterfly.

When she grew from bean to big enough for me to feel her every turn and kick, I knew I was going to be in for it. She kicked often and hard. Even when my belly grew quiet and her movements slowed down, it wasn't long before a swift kick reminded me that she was here, strong and determined. There was something about those kicks that already felt familiar. I knew this girl. I had a feeling that she would be busy. We were healthy, but the shadow of the crash remained, and this time it reached Scott.

A week before we were scheduled to go to the hospital to deliver our daughter, Scott and I were about to attend a service at church, when he stopped to chat with a neighbor in the parking lot. I waited at the doors until he joined me. "I feel like I can't breathe," he said. "I think you need to take me to a clinic."

"What? Are you serious?"

"Yeah. Something is wrong. I can't see straight. I need to go. Now."

We got into the car, and I drove him to the clinic. Bewildered, I didn't understand what was happening, but I was confident he would be fine.

He wasn't fine.

He had a panic attack and began to unravel. Earlier, Scott had been told we'd have to put in thirteen thousand dollars of work toward sewage for our home. His mind began to spin and he was powerless to stop it. How would he come up with that money? Later, he learned it wasn't true, and the neighbor got it wrong. It was for *their* home, not ours. But that large sum was dropped into Scott's lap, and he snapped.

He was overcome with anxiety and a mind racing ninety miles an hour. He had seen his doctor and made an appointment to see a counselor. Scott was here, but not *here*, and I felt alone. The rest of the week was a blur. We had a baby coming, and I couldn't concentrate on what was happening to the steadfast Scott I knew. He was unable to carry a conversation without extreme anxiety, often stopping mid-thought and abruptly going silent.

He appeared lost, and I didn't know how to help. I couldn't help. I didn't know what *this* was. I told myself we were experiencing a hiccup, a bump in the road. He's having a bad week. There's a lot going on. The money he thought he'd have to pay, the baby, another surgery, and returning to the hospital. I was sure that after we had our daughter, Scott would come back.

The doctor said that once Scott saw the counselor, we would get some answers. Until then, the doctor prescribed Ativan (a medicine to help treat anxiety) to get him through our baby's birth a week later.

"Are you okay?" I asked as we were about to go into surgery to have our baby. Scott was here, doing and saying all the right things, but he felt far away. He had used the word breakdown the night before and I responded with denial. *Are you sure?* I treaded lightly. Maybe we were making too big a deal out of this. Maybe this was just a very bad week. It's what I wanted to believe. All I could think about was having this baby and my need for him. We were going to be parents. Maybe the birth of our baby girl would shed new light and bring an end to all that was going on.

"I'm okay. Don't worry about me. I've got my pills. Let's have our daughter."

He wore a hospital-issued gown and mask that covered his mouth and nose, but I could see his eyes clearly. What I saw startled me. I had been so busy preparing and packing for our baby and our hospital stay, I didn't see him. He was barely holding it together. He wasn't okay. Breakdown hung between us. This was a shattered man.

Fear lurched and suddenly stopped. I couldn't do this right now, and I told myself to calm down and get ready to have a baby.

There was a curtain between my head and pregnant belly. Scott sat near my head. Our doctor asked if he wanted to cut the umbilical cord after our baby was born. "No. I'm good right here." We had already discussed how he would stay behind the curtain. He was squeamish about blood and he didn't want to see me cut open. This felt normal. This is the Scott I know.

There is nothing unusual about him wanting to stay close to my face, but…he took a pill. He never had to take anything to see me in the burn unit. He was never unsteady on his feet like he was today. He had never felt so far away, and it scared me. Maybe all the years of holding it together since the crash had taken its toll. I didn't know what was happening, but whatever this was, I knew I couldn't deny it anymore. He was slipping away from me, and I didn't know how to stop it. I reached for Scott's hand as the anesthetic slipped through my spine and froze half my body. Nausea rippled through me and I waited for the cry of my baby.

~~~

Annie Elizabeth, named after Betty (Elisabeth Anne), was lifted from me by C-section on July 4, 2003. My pregnancy had been a time of worry. Ultrasounds showed markers for Down's syndrome, she was too small and there wasn't enough amniotic fluid, and in spite of all the dark clouds, she was born perfectly healthy, bald and blue-eyed. I had yearned for her, and she became my redemption.

I marveled at her legs, her feet, and her soft, unmarked skin. It was humbling that she came new and whole from my beaten and battered body. While I loved her and curled myself around her small soft body, I had feelings I didn't anticipate. I wasn't taken with her immediately, like I was promised. I didn't know if it was an offshoot from my worrying about Scott, or post-partum depression, but the earth didn't move, the heavens didn't open, and I didn't find my calling in my child. Instead, I was plunged into motherhood wholly unprepared.

It didn't matter that I had spent a lot of time with other moms, or read books, or fantasized about my baby in cute clothes. I felt guilty of not feeling warm and fuzzy like a Hallmark card, of which I had bought many to congratulate new mothers on their adorable new bundles. There was no question of my love for this tiny wrinkled being, it was the "forever" part that hit home. It didn't help when I came up from my C-section stupor and a nurse put her to my breast and said, "She's hungry."

The evening after I'd had Annie, she fussed and cried, and I couldn't get that latch right. A nurse decided this would be the perfect time to remind me of the huge changes I was about to embrace. "Your life isn't yours anymore. It is all about her now."

Dread filled me, and shame wasn't far behind. *Shouldn't this be good news? This should make me happy.* I wanted the parenting magazine face, that blissful, serene face that reflected how I worshiped the miracle in my arms. Instead, my face was lined with fear and anxiety.

It was still difficult to be on my feet, in my legs for long periods of time, so my body was prone to fatigue and skin breakdown. I used to be able to rest and take off my legs and lounge on the couch for a while to give my legs and skin a break.

Having Annie gave me a new schedule, and my body had to adjust to it fast. I had many needs, and now I had a baby who also had needs. My fatigue reached new heights, and I felt as though I was in shock, sleep-deprived shock. I thought if I willed it, I could be contented. We would go out, just the two of us! And I'd prove I could be a good mom.

I thought I knew what I was getting into, and knew my world would be filled with diapers and sleep deprivation. Mothers laughed about this over cups of coffee as they hugged their babies close to them. No one mentioned the guilt I now felt as a new mom, and how coffee was a lifeline, the only thing that made me feel human after a restless night.

We had planned for Annie, not that I could use that as an excuse for my feelings. There would be rationale in a surprise pregnancy, but we had wanted and loved her before she was conceived, and that love expanded and grew twice its size when I realized she was on her way.

I had spent years working to make my life predictable and even. Bouncing a baby on my hip threw my life for another loop, and I never saw it coming.

Annie was a few weeks old when I decided to take her out for more than a doctor's visit. A friend was visiting from out of town and it was the perfect excuse for a girls' night. Annie, sound asleep, was bundled and scrunched in her car seat as our group of friends caught up. Talk turned to me, the brand new mom. How was it going?

All eyes were on me. "She's a good sleeper. I mean, I'm up with her a lot, but she sleeps pretty well, I think. She wants to nurse a lot, and, well, I don't love breastfeeding." *There. I said it.* "But I'm doing it anyway because it's good for her," I added quickly, absolving myself.

I attempted more honesty, trying to articulate how I felt, even though I didn't understand how I felt. "I love Annie. I do. I just feel like I haven't really bonded with her yet." I looked around the table, hoping for reassuring words and smiles. I respected my friends who had already blazed this mom trail. Maybe they would have some wise advice for me, or their own tales of breastfeeding woes and conflicted feelings. My admission was met with silence. Flooded with shame, I scrambled to make up for what I'd just said.

"I'm sure it will get better. I'm just new to all of this."

I looked around the table at their blank faces and felt my face grow hot with humiliation. Was I alone in these feelings? I couldn't be the only one who felt insecure.

My girls' night out proved to be more frustrating than enlightening. Instead of hearing a chorus of "Me, too," I'd been met with blank stares and silence, as if I was some kind of anomaly who was unfit for motherhood. I couldn't tell them about Scott, either, so I felt alone.

My feelings of inadequacy and frustration didn't end there. Not only was I a new mom, but I realized I was still learning a new normal. It had been five years since the crash, and I thought I was doing well. But the additional strain on my body and legs catapulted me to the past. Now it seemed Scott was coming undone. Caught in the echoes of the crash, we felt the fire and the loss of my skin and limbs all over again. Taking care of Annie would be easier if I was able-bodied. When she cried in the night, I fumbled with my prostheses until I got them on. I couldn't simply reach for her to feed her. I needed feet to prop myself up and hold her in the right position. Frustrated that I couldn't move faster, I hated that she had to wait for me to pick her up, or that I had to ask Scott for help. I should be able to do this. Could I give her all that she needs?

Scott was helpful, even in his fog. He changed her diapers, rocked her to sleep, and cradled her in his arms. He gave me breaks when I needed them, encouraging me to lie down or get out of the house for a while. In his fragile mental state, he found looking after Annie soothing. It wasn't complicated to button her pajamas or pat her back, and this comforted him. He was an attentive father. But I was very aware that we were just surviving again. While survival was familiar, and it had been proven we were good under pressure, what was going on with Scott was something new, something we didn't understand yet.

I couldn't do much for him except be there for him like he had been there for me. One evening, after seeing his counselor, he came home and said, "So it looks like I'm depressed. I've probably been depressed for a long time."

And as he explained the depression, how he was tormented by anxiety, my suspicion was confirmed. The breakdown he suffered weeks ago was about the lingering effects of the car crash. The crash had been a trigger. It seemed Scott had been depressed long before the crash, and his calm demeanor masked his feelings of hopelessness. I hadn't known Scott that long when I landed in the hospital, so I didn't notice how often he found the world flat, not round with possibility. He had always been quiet and reserved and had never been one to discuss his feelings at great length. Scott was also unaware of his depression and believed the way he thought and felt were normal, just "who he is." When the crash happened, he swung into superhero mode, busy with saving and rescuing. But something inside him began to crack. This was big, and the hurt couldn't be contained. He had been traumatized like I had been traumatized. His counselor talked to him about coping skills, triggers, and dealing with his emotions.

At home, there was routine, and Scott seemed at ease there. He had his own business, so his time was flexible. When work overwhelmed him, he could come home to rest. But going out and seeing friends caused his anxiety to escalate, so he stayed home, and I made excuses for him. It was hard to explain to people how he found conversation and noise crippling. He buried himself in sleep and silence. I hardly understood what was going on with him. I wanted to shake him, to yell where did you go? And drag him back from "over there." But I didn't. I couldn't. I had to be careful. Life was too much for him.

Again, I saw how little control we had over our world, how life could change in an instant, and I pushed down my fear. I wanted to be a haven for him, someone safe as he defined depression. I listened and gave him space when he needed to be alone. I promised I'd be there and tried to be understanding. In order to keep things calm, I tiptoed around him. At the same time, I was wound tight and still overcome with all that I couldn't do.

It got harder to separate Scott from depression. Depression greeted me at the door when I came home. It was on the couch. In my bed. It was everywhere, all the time, stale and lonely. All I could offer was space and feeble, but sincere, attempts at help. Are you okay? What can I do? Nothing. I couldn't do anything. I gave him more space. I had Annie to take care of.

As Scott worked on himself, I worked on my new role. Being a mom was not something I could pick up or put down on a whim. I was on call all the time. My baby and my body were demanding and high maintenance. I had to adapt. Again. Bit by bit I adjusted to our changing world until the distance between us diminished, and she was a part of me, my daughter.

Hearing Annie giggle for the first time was the sweetest sound I'd ever heard. I didn't know a heart could explode with love like that, and I did everything in my power to coax that giggle from her again and again. One afternoon after a fussy, busy morning I leaned over her bassinet and stroked the soft curve of her rosy cheek, hot with the sleep she had finally succumbed to, and I thought *I get it*. A mother's love. I had come a long way to meet this girl, and the fact that she was here at all was its own miracle. As Annie and I got closer and I became more confident in my ability to take care of her, I could turn more of my attention to Scott.

He saw the counselor once a week, and after many months of meeting with him, they decided he should go on anti-depressants.

"Do you think this is the answer?" I asked. "Will this help you?"

"I don't know if it's *the* answer, but it's *an* answer," Scott said. "My brain is squirrely... it feels broken. I need help coping. The crash really tipped me over the edge. I've given it a lot of thought, and I'm going to try it. If it doesn't work, we'll figure it out."

I didn't know how to feel. Would the medication change him? Would he still be the man I married? Would he always need it? And did that matter? If it helped, I decided it didn't matter. The light in him had been snuffed out, and I missed him.

I hoped it would work. I needed for it to work.

Our lives changed again, and this time, for the better. Over the next month, I saw Scott emerge. He was still my Scott, with a dry sense of humor and that evenness I loved. But it was also a Scott with a clearer head and skills to cope. He confronted his suppressed grief and talked to me about it, finally letting me in. He told me every time he heard the phone ring unexpectedly there was a flashback to the life-changing phone call he received, and it rattled him as he relived the heartache of that evening. I saw hints of hope and optimism as he complained less and joked more about his squirrely brain. His stomach wasn't as twisted and tied up anymore. There was light in his eyes again. He still struggled with anxiety, but he began to grasp his limits and knew to tell me if he had to retreat when the day had been too much.

As our family began to stabilize, I could breathe again. I knew depression was around, not far away, but my fear that we would always live in the shadow of the crash weakened. I longed to move beyond it and thrive.

~~~

Two years after the trial, two years after a judge sentenced Jeff to one year in prison, guilty of dangerous driving causing bodily harm and dangerous driving causing death, I happened to be flipping through channels on TV, when a trial on the news caught my eye.

A man had been found guilty of the murders of many women, and he stood in court to listen to the families' testimonies of how he had ripped their lives apart.

He stood silently, a stone wall, hearing people's grief spill over him. Many cried and raged, and some interrupted with whispers of forgiveness. The camera panned over to the man, the killer, the stone wall. The only time he flinched was when the words, "I forgive you" found their way to him.

I watched the man's face on my TV screen intently. Again I heard, "I forgive you." Stirred by his expression, the twist in his features as people spoke with grace, compassion bloomed in my belly. Jeff flashed in my mind. I never felt the need to forgive Jeff, even when he turned to face us in court. Now, watching the change in this murderer's face, I was drawn to forgiveness. Was this something I needed to do? My compassion for Jeff astonished me.

Sunday school lessons taught me about turning the other cheek, that forgiveness was a way of life. While some of Betty's family members forgave, I couldn't. I didn't want my reason for forgiving Jeff to be due to religion or because I was raised to be a good girl. If I forgave, it should be real and from the heart.

Something awakened inside me, something I hadn't been aware of mattering until this moment. I wasn't sure that I needed to forgive Jeff in order to move on. After all, I was busy living and didn't feel held back. I was careful with my thoughts around Jeff. Any emotion that surfaced after the trial and sentencing was squashed.

He could not have room in my life again. I had met people fixated on revenge and saw how their anger devoured them. I swore that wouldn't be me, and I wouldn't be the person blinded by bitterness. After sentencing, I wanted to be free of him, and being free of him meant not thinking about him, or wasting any energy on him.

Maybe forgiving him would be true freedom. I wore the marks of the crash, of his choices, every day. But maybe today I'd get rid of his residue, the scars that lined my soul, and finally purge him.

I wondered if Jeff's mind and face and heart would change, too, if I offered forgiveness. And if it didn't do anything, if he stayed the same, would I still forgive? My stomach fluttered again, and I knew this new mercy stemmed from the heart. My heart hadn't led me astray yet, so I trusted my heart and decided I wanted to forgive.

I could not ignore what was happening to me on this ordinary afternoon in my living room, with my baby. The desire swelled, and I knew I had to set him free, and in doing so, I'd set myself free. This wasn't about absolving him; he was guilty. But I needed to let him go. It was time. I was angry at his sentencing, and now...now I wanted peace. I believed in peace. The right time found me.

I wiped tears from my eyes as I looked at my daughter gurgling and rosy-cheeked on the floor. I picked her up, and she burrowed her face into my neck. Life was short. I knew that all too well.

I whispered, "I forgive you," to Annie, to the room, to Jeff. Immediately, I felt lighter, as my burden lifted, and a new desire took its place, one that surprised me.

That evening I told Scott about my out-of-the-blue encounter with forgiveness. "I think I might want to get in touch with Jeff if it's possible. I just want to see him and forgive out loud, you know? What do you think? Do you think it's a bad idea?"

Scott was quiet for a few seconds. I waited while he put on his thinking face. He was careful with his words, always contemplating before he spoke. "No. I don't think it's a bad idea. I get what you want to do and understand why. Just be prepared that it might not go the way you hope. What do you hope for?"

"I'm not sure exactly. I know I don't want to rake over the past. I just want to see him and say the words, I forgive you."

"Will it matter to you if he doesn't care? He might not want to see you."

"I don't know," I said truthfully. "I haven't thought that far ahead. I just feel I have to try." This was a rash decision, but once I made up my mind it was hard to change.

"Then you should try."

I got in touch with the mediator who helped Betty's family. We eventually connected through email, and I asked if it would be possible to meet with Jeff.

The mediator, Charles, wasn't sure. The conditions of Jeff's sentence were long over and even though he was on parole, he was under no obligation to meet with me. He met with Betty's family and fulfilled that part of his sentence.

I assured Charles that I harbored no ill will toward Jeff and had no desire to rehash the past. This wasn't going to be about ranting and raving. I wanted to see Jeff, to look him in the eye and say *I forgive you* and hope he would go on to lead a happy life.

I waited, nervous Jeff would say yes, and nervous he would say no. What would it be like to meet him, to speak to him? What I wanted was one-sided; I didn't want to hear from him. I wasn't after an apology or an explanation. Our lives were horribly joined together, and I wanted to cut myself loose. Like the man with cracks in the stone wall, I hoped my forgiveness would stir Jeff and set him free, set both of us free. I knew this wouldn't wipe out what he had done. There would be days where anger reared its head, and forgiveness would be a choice, a daily exercise of letting go. I didn't know if he deserved a second chance, but redemption was possible for anyone.

The mediator emailed me after a few days. "I'm sorry, Heidi. He wants to move forward with his life and put the past behind him."

Disappointment settled over me, gray and muddy, and suddenly it wasn't a want anymore. This desire to see him had grown into need. Scott's words echoed in my ear. What if he doesn't care? At the time, I didn't know how I would feel. I believed that no matter the outcome, I would be fine. But I had begun to care about Jeff's response. I wanted him to care, to care enough to see me. If I had hurt someone and there was an opportunity for grace, I would lunge for it. I didn't understand him, and I had to remind myself that making him care wasn't my original intent. It was about peace. My peace.

He had asked for forgiveness in court, and I did not lift my head to meet his eyes. This time I wanted to look him in the eyes and simply say yes. If I couldn't see him, I'd put the words on paper and send forgiveness to him.

I asked Charles, "Could I write him a letter?"

"I'll do my best to get it to him, but I can't make any promises."

For days I expressed my forgiveness and wished him well. I wrote and rewrote my heart on paper. *You don't have to be tied to me anymore.* To forgive was to let him go.

I sealed the envelope, almost certain I wouldn't hear from him, but hoped that maybe I was wrong. Either way, I knew I needed to do this, and I felt peace wash over me as I dropped the letter into the mailbox. It was better to let go than to hang on.

I never heard from him.

29
Whole

I wasn't scaling mountains. I wasn't jumping out of planes.

I *could* finally watch a romantic comedy without being irritated with the girl who was beautiful but didn't know it, or the girl who worked hard and needed to make room for romance with the guy who had been there all along. I could take care of someone else other than me. I could feel pretty again.

I learned how to live life with a disability until disability wasn't as obvious, so *there*. I used to wear shorts for purely practical reasons, the ease of taking my legs on and off, but as I got better and stronger, I wore pants. I learned to dress myself again, finding pants and jeans that fit over bulky legs. I wanted to be pretty, to look like everyone else, to wear cute clothes and not functional ones. I was fussy and high-maintenance with skin to lotion each day, legs to put on, and appointments that lasted hours.

My former orderly's words of deliverance found their way to me once more. Denny had told me, "You need to feel like a girl again." I did need it, and I pursued that need. It wasn't just about reaching out to that twenty-three year old girl, but embracing a twenty-six year old woman who was growing up and wanted to keep up with the women around her. I wanted to blend in, and it pleased me so much when I did.

If my not-so-secret was discovered, "You're an amputee?!" Pride would color my answer, "Yeah, I am."

Their eyes would do a quick once over to take inventory. "You can't tell!" I was like everyone else, just with metal parts.

I also recognized that sometimes I wasn't like everyone else.

I continually forged a relationship with my scars. I would be in this body, in this skin for a long time, and for a long time I wished I could shed it, wriggle out of it. But this was my body, and I wanted to serve it like it had served me. I had found beauty when I didn't think it was mine to have, and I would uncover it again.

While I didn't love my scars, I called a truce with them, acknowledging they were a map of where I'd been and how hard I'd fought.

There was a slow and subtle shift in my worry about my legs feeling foreign. After I got new prosthetics, they fit better and hugged my legs. They became less like a pair of ill-fitting boots, and more a part of me.

There was a perk to having prosthetic legs; I got to pick my foot size. My feet used to be a size eight, and I decided to switch it up with size sevens. I liked the idea of having smaller feet, and why not? I had grown to appreciate my prosthetics. They weren't going anywhere. I relied on them to get me around. They became my legs because they had to be. They joined me, and I them.

So when the skin on my legs broke down, and I was in and out of my prosthetist's office often, I was frustrated. I liked Dana, but neither of us needed to see each other this much.

My first prosthetist, David, had affectionately called me The Princess and the Pea. I noticed everything amiss.

One leg could be a little shorter than the other, hitching up my hip as I walked, so Dana lowered or lengthened my prosthetics until I wasn't walking around like Frankenstein. If my legs had calves that looked too fat, Dana obliged me and scaled them down. If I was pigeon-toed he'd fix that. Not much escaped him. As soon as I walked through the door with the slightest limp, he'd see it, or notice a mark that was just too red on my leg. As tired as I was of going to see him, he was my leg guy, and I depended on him.

Chronic pain accompanied the broken skin that came from constant chafing from my prosthetic leg. This was only the beginning, and I learned skin breakdown would be something I would always struggle with because of the damage done by fire. I played the game of Catch-22 with my legs. My skin needed air and rest to get better, but I needed to be able to get around, so I couldn't afford the time to give it air and rest. I healed at a snail's pace too, so when skin came apart, it was a laborious journey to get better.

The back and forth of it was exhausting, and the pain begat misery. I accepted and made peace, but my skin was making it hard to maintain my good will.

Dana knew me well. "This is getting to you. You usually come in smiling."

"I'm frustrated, Dana. I know you're doing everything you can. My skin just sucks."

"You're tired."

I smiled weakly. "I am."

"We'll figure it out, Heidi."

Dana was just as committed as I was to my vision of normal life.

This was my new normal—balancing appointments, a beat-up body, being a wife and mother. Yet somewhere in between all this, I somehow managed to stave off misery and began to do more than survive. I began to live.

Time created a gap between me and the crash. Life overcame loss until it wasn't just about the trial or what happened in the ravine. While my broken skin was a serious problem, there were moments, even days of reprieve, and I didn't look at myself in the mirror and feel haunted by what had been. I didn't see every flaw and pieces that were missing. I fully owned who and what I wanted to be.

I could place as much or as little emphasis as I wanted on being a survivor and amputee. There was no doubt that the crash changed me. In a split second, it claimed me and shaped me, but it wasn't *all* of me. I didn't stick out my hand when I met someone new and introduce myself as a burn survivor and double amputee. I was just like everyone else; I'd do just about anything for a particular food I craved, I was opinionated and stubborn, and believed in more for my life. I had love and knew love. I found my version of whole.

I was what I longed to be, what I had fought for—ordinary. I was just a girl, just a woman with hope and dreams and a life.

30
Thank You for Saving Me

"Heidi, I have a favor to ask you. A pretty big favor. You can say no."

"Okay..."

It was my friend, Karen. "I'm thinking of putting on a concert for Vancouver. I want it to be a community thing, and I'd like to give the proceeds to the burn fund. I was wondering if you could speak at the concert. Tell your story. It would be on behalf of the burn fund."

"Oh, um, okay. Well, let me think about it."

"Of course! Think about it. Take all the time you need and get back to me."

Karen was easy like that. No big deal, take your time, and you can change your mind.

I got off the phone and looked at Scott, who was sitting on the couch next to me. "Do you know Karen's putting on a concert? She wants me to speak. It'll be for the burn fund."

"Do you want to do it?"

"Not really, but I might do it for Karen. And it's for the burn fund."

I had been cautious about telling my story. Karen hadn't been the first person to ask. Various people had asked me to tell my story for various audiences—high school students, inspirational groups. I'd been so intent on getting on with my life that I worried about being dragged under by rehashing my story at such a vulnerable time. I also felt it was too intimate to take people into my pain, exposing myself on a stage or behind a microphone. I knew the point wasn't the pain, but the triumph, the overcoming. The surviving. The British Columbia Professional Firefighters Burn Fund promoted survivors. They had a significant impact on how I viewed my life.

I never wanted to be the poster girl for burn survivors because I'd fought so hard to be ordinary, someone who blended with society. I knew many people became advocates after they'd suffered cancer, collision, or disease, but I didn't necessarily like the idea that I had to do something just because I was in a car crash. I wanted to amount to something, *be* something, not because I was burnt or my legs were cut off, but because I was being myself.

It had been seven years since the crash, and I still felt as though I was on a detour, and that one day I would get myself back on track. Isn't that what people said? Except I kept wondering, what track?

I wasn't on a track. I hadn't even picked a track. I couldn't return *to* anything. At twenty-three, I was at the age of figuring things out, of destiny-making. At thirty, I still didn't know what lay ahead. I had spent such a long time in recovery, got married, had a baby, and now I was expecting another baby. And nowhere along the way had I discovered what I *should* be doing, if there was anything to do at all. All my life I'd heard the question, *what are you passionate about?* That was easy; I was passionate about living.

It looked like my fate was finding me. Maybe telling my story was part of my destiny. I could say no and be fine, or I could risk it and go public. I could be a reluctant storyteller telling her story, but what would it lead to? I couldn't be sure. I was afraid and excited all at the same time. Maybe for five minutes I could be an ordinary woman telling her extraordinary story. And it would be good to give back.

Five minutes after Karen's phone call, I called her back. "I'll do it."

That's how the World Service concert was born. The concert would be held in May of 2005 at the Pacific Coliseum in Vancouver, and the purpose was to give to the community and serve the burn fund like it had served the city. People would buy tickets to see the concert, allowing that some of the proceeds would cover the costs of putting on the show, and the rest would go to the burn fund. World Service would raise money to buy a piece of high-tech equipment for the Burns and Plastics unit.

It was important to Karen to do this right, and she began to gather a team of people to help assemble and sponsor the event. One of the things she wanted to do was create a short five minute documentary. Scott, my friend, Angela, the police at the scene, and the firefighters were interviewed to assist in telling my story and showing various stages of my recovery through a compilation of photos. I came in, too, serving as narrator.

There was one more thing—we needed photos from the scene of the crash. I braced myself for the onslaught of emotion. Returning to that day wouldn't be easy, no matter how much time had passed.

~~~

I met Detective Kevin Wright at his office. The building was buzzing with activity when I arrived, so he pulled the door shut and opened the file on his desk. There weren't just a few photos. There was a stack of them. He looked uncomfortable as he looked at me. "You don't want to see all of these. There are some you just shouldn't see."

He pulled out the photos and asked if I was okay, if I was ready to see them.

The first one I saw was of my car in the ravine. It was red, twisted, squished, a jumble of metal.

Breathe in and out. It's going to be okay. I am all right.

The next one I saw was of me being pulled from the car. Hands supporting me, I was on my back. My jeans hung from me, my legs exposed. Red, raw, damaged. My eyes open.

"Are you okay?"

"Yup. I'm fine." I smiled, trying to convince him and me. I crossed my arms to hold myself still. I pinched the skin of the soft underside of my arm to keep from crying.

My eyes were open in those photos. My undoing, my horror witnessed on film, and I couldn't recall a second of it. I had been told I was conscious when I was rescued, and the proof lay in front of me.

My eyes were open when I was on fire, when I was trapped, when Betty lay still beside me.

He handed me a few pictures of the mangled car and kept the ones of me in his hand. I was relieved not to see any of Betty. I preferred to keep her image intact, of her smiling and happy, whole.

Eager to move away from the heartbreak of the photos, I asked him how he was doing, and what he'd been up to.

He smiled. "I think that's something I should be asking you."

My burst of honesty surprised me. "After looking at those photos, I don't know what to say. It's a lot harder than I thought it would be."

As we caught up on our lives and families, I was astonished at all that I'd accomplished in the seven years since the crash, how far I'd come and how long I'd been removed from the "old" me. Finally, I was alive, truly alive, and seeing the evidence of death and being reminded of that split second of fate left me shaken. I needed a little time to recover.

I hugged Kevin goodbye and left the station, where I could take refuge in my car. I tucked the photos in my bag and put it on the floor of the passenger side, nudging it with my foot to move it as far away from me as possible. As I turned up the music and drove down the road, I let my tears fall, finding solace in the loudness, in the rain that fell hard on my windshield, in the swish of the wipers.

~~~

I didn't see the video footage until after the interviews were shot. I was asked to take a look at the rough cut.

In a room alone with the computer, I watched each interview and each photo unfold on the screen. I arrived at the part where the firefighters were interviewed. Standing serious and tall, they were emotional as they told their stories.

I realized I didn't know their names, these men who had saved my life. They spoke of getting the call, of coming down, of assessing the damage, of throwing down hoses, of my cries for help.

The car was upside down, sinking further into the shallow water at the bottom of the ravine. They sprayed the car to put out the fire and cool me off. A firefighter held my hand as they prepared to pry me out. After all the noise and chaos, after the Jaws of Life were used to extract me, after I was lifted into an ambulance, this amazing firefighter stayed with me for a while, in the aftermath, in the quiet.

In front of me were my heroes in uniform: Capt. Larry Hooge, John Markwat, Capt. Ken Nickel, and Deputy Chief Dale Unrau.

The paramedic made sure to tell my parents that I was calm in the ambulance. She was surprised by my politeness, since she was used to more colorful language when transporting people to the hospital. Over and over again, I stated, "This is awful," and she wanted to meet the parents of this girl, to tell them they must have raised me right.

My mom was home when it happened, and I can only imagine her horror. It was just after eight in the evening and she had returned from grocery shopping. She heard the crash, loud, *like a bomb went off*, she explained to police officers later. Betty and I had left only seconds ago.

She ran out of the house, toward the main intersection, toward the sound and smoke. Cars pulled over; people climbed out of their vehicles and raced from their homes. The fence across the street was torn down. A car she didn't recognize was up against the curb by the remains of the fence.

Frantic, she asked everyone, "Did you see a red car with two girls in it?"

A neighbor called 911.

Two men climbed down the ravine to find out for her. Neighbors gathered and murmured prayers as my mom waited.

One of the men returned. "It's a red car! There are two girls in it."

Shawn, the other man, remained at the bottom of the ravine where my car had landed upside down and was on fire. I was in the car screaming, "What happened?"

He wanted to help, to do something. Risking his own safety, he reached for Betty through the smashed window and felt for her pulse. He couldn't find one. He came around to my side and tried to undo my seat belt. It wouldn't budge. Worried about smoke inhalation, he stretched my neck and head out the window. I had tied a sweater around my waist which flipped and hung over my face, acting as a flimsy shield.

I begged Shawn, "Please don't leave me." He assured me he wasn't going anywhere.

Police, at the top of the ravine, were yelling for him to come up. It was too dangerous for him to be there.

He yelled back, "I made a promise!" He cradled my head in his hands while his boots melted from the heat of the fire.

Somebody handed my mom a cell phone. The only number that came to her mind was my brother, Ron, who made more calls to family.

Betty's family needed to know, but my mom couldn't bring herself to call, uncertain whether she could speak Betty's name into the phone. The family had already seen so much tragedy. With Betty's mother being killed in a crash, and now her daughter, how could she be the one to inflict this pain? Someone else reached them.

Sirens wailing, the firefighters arrived and began their rescue amidst my cries, begging for God to answer…

~~~

I wrapped my arms around my body, holding myself in as I saw the snapshots of me smiling, young, happy in Hawaii, then my mangled car, sick in a hospital bed, standing on my prosthetic legs for the first time, of me and Angela, her arm around me in the hospital bed, Angela calmly telling her story, Scott telling his story, police officer interviews, and firefighters' interviews.

I vibrated with memories and was flooded with new knowledge of the horror of that day. The firefighters' recount of the crash filled in the gaps for me. These were pieces I hadn't heard yet.

It rattled me to hear my story from others' point of view, to see pain twist their faces while speaking in hushed voices about how helpless we were, trapped and waiting. It was a lot to bear. I took the facts in with my mind, but it was my body that manifested the trauma. My trembling limbs gave away how my life changed that day. In a split second, I would never be the same.

Edited to five minutes over music and sirens, the video bore witness to Betty's and my undoing, my recovery, and ended with the day I got married.

While the video went into editing, I set out to write my five minute speech. I was given a lot of advice, like don't write it out, but just speak from the heart. I would be standing in front of two thousand people, so yes, I would write the speech. From the heart.

~~~

The day of the concert, Scott and I went into the city early, caught a movie, and headed to the Coliseum. As we drove toward the entrance I saw my name wink and flash on the huge black screen.

I grabbed Scott's arm. "There's my name! My name! In lights. Can you believe it?" I was embarrassed, delighted, and then nauseous. "My name is up there. In lights. I think I'm going to throw up."

It was a long day. I walked around the coliseum and saw the stage I'd be standing on, then I did a television interview for a Vancouver news station in the afternoon, followed by a radio interview in the evening. I talked about the importance of the event, how the burn fund and firefighters saved my life, and how they are truly heroes.

I was a fit of nerves in the minutes preceding my speech, and there was no convincing my hands to warm up and stop shaking. I waited beside the stage in the dark when I remembered there were stairs leading up to the stage.

Why didn't I anticipate stairs? I'd thought through everything, so how did I miss this? I was seized with a familiar feeling of panic. I would be too slow climbing them. What if I don't get onto the stage fast enough? What if there is a long uncomfortable silence while I lumber up the stairs, everyone hearing my footsteps?

After thirty seconds of gut-wrenching anxiety I realized it didn't matter if I was slow. It would only feel that way to me. I took a deep breath.

The band wrapped up their set, which meant the big screen would soon light up with the five minute video of my story.

Two thousand people filled the stadium and I had never spoken to a crowd this large. The video played, flashing all the faces who had a big hand in my survival and recovery. I tried hard not to cry, but I couldn't reign myself in. I needed to speak in a minute and the tears kept coming. I pressed both hands to my cheeks, trying to hold myself together. *You can do this.*

I walked up the stairs, holding onto the railing.

The video came to an end. A beat of silence.

The presenter said, "Ladies and Gentlemen! Heidi Cave!"

I stepped onto the stage into the bright lights above me. People stood and clapped. I continued to cry, awash in light and applause. I wiped my eyes, took a shaky breath, and let my voice fill the coliseum. The final highlight of the evening was helping present a check of twenty thousand dollars to the Burn Fund.

Three months later, I gave birth to Benjamin. There was so much to live for.

Acknowledgements

Thank you to my agent Elizabeth Kracht for asking me to dig deep and giving me the best advice ever—to say what I mean. Also, thank you for calling me energetic when I worried about being a crazy author lady. You are a joy. Thank you to my editor, Lynn Price, who let me pitch my story to her just before dinner and just before all of us were too into the wine. Thank you for your faith in me and your quick replies. I reached depths I didn't know were possible because of you and your lay-it-on-the-line notes.

I'm so grateful to my early readers Jo, Scott R, Jordan and Jenn for your feedback, honesty and help. Oh, the help! For this, and your friendship, thank you.

Thank you to the girls who have been there before the beginning. Ang: for "getting" me and never letting me give up even when I really wanted to. Loraleigh: who sees more for me than I do. Tanya: who truly listens and understands the importance of treats.

I can't list all of my dear friends who have encouraged me and believed in me. It would go on for pages. Thank you, with all my heart.

Thanks to my short-lived but much appreciated writers group for challenging me with more. More, more, more. I still hear it in my head when I write.

A heartfelt holla to the ladies at PNWA (you know who you are) who went out of their way to make sure I wasn't a wallflower.

When I began to try out this story, worrying and wondering if I was doing the right thing, I was fortunate to have my very own online cheerleaders. I am so grateful for the people who read my blog, who came alongside me and my story. Many have become friends. Thank you for being in my corner.

Danke to my parents, Theodor and Trudy, for loving me unconditionally. Dad, thank you for teaching me generosity by example. Mom, you are one of the strongest people I know. You are my backbone. Big thanks to my brothers, Ron and Rick, who are always genuinely happy for me.

Not everyone can say they have great in-laws, but I can, and I mean it. Thank you for your love, support, and telling everyone, including most of Quesnel, about *Fancy Feet*.

Thank you to Detective Kevin Wright for answering my questions and giving me the background to the background. Thank you to my fire fighters, the incredible staff at the Vancouver General Hospital burn unit and G.F. Strong, Tony Burke, and the BC Professional Fire Fighters burn fund for making me a survivor. Without you, there wouldn't be a story to tell.

When I ran out of words, music and books helped fill the quiet, inspiring me to keep writing. There are far too many artists and authors to list here, but I am completely serious when I say that I owe music and books huge.

Annie and Benjamin, the best kids in the world. You are my reason.

Scott, this memoir wouldn't have happened without you. I'm so glad we decided to do life together.

Betty, you're in a book! For the too short time you lived here, a light on the earth, you made my life warmer and sweeter. I want you to know you live on here in the minds and hearts of the people who love you. Beautiful, beautiful Betty.